Doing a
Research Project *in*
Nursing & Midwifery

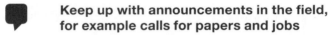
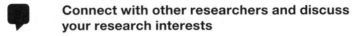
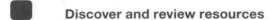
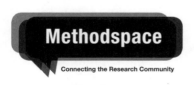
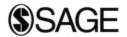

Doing a Research Project in Nursing & Midwifery

A Basic Guide to Research Using the Literature Review Methodology

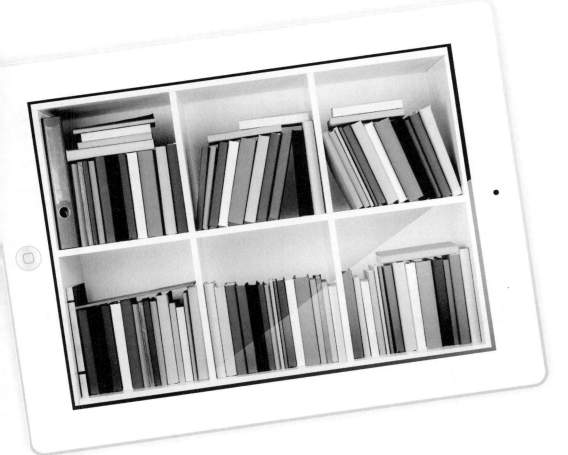

Los Angeles | London | New Delhi
Singapore | Washington DC

Carroll Siu
and Huguette Comerasamy

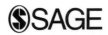

Los Angeles | London | New Delhi
Singapore | Washington DC

SAGE Publications Ltd
1 Oliver's Yard
55 City Road
London EC1Y 1SP

SAGE Publications Inc.
2455 Teller Road
Thousand Oaks, California 91320

SAGE Publications India Pvt Ltd
B 1/I 1 Mohan Cooperative Industrial Area
Mathura Road
New Delhi 110 044

SAGE Publications Asia-Pacific Pte Ltd
3 Church Street
#10-04 Samsung Hub
Singapore 049483

Editor: Katie Metzler
Assistant Editor: Anna Horvai
Copyeditor: Sarah Bury
Proofreader: Derek Markham
Marketing manager: Tamara Navaratnam
Cover design: Francis Kenney
Typeset by: C&M Digitals (P) Ltd, Chennai, India
Printed by: MPG Printgroup, UK

Library of Congress Control Number: 2012944106

British Library Cataloguing in Publication data

A catalogue record for this book is available from
the British Library

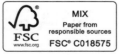

MIX
Paper from
responsible sources
FSC
www.fsc.org FSC® C018575

ISBN 978-0-85702-747-4
ISBN 978-0-85702-748-1 (pbk)

To our students

Contents

List of Tables

List of Figures

Authors

Carroll King Ling Siu (RGN, RM, RNT, BSc in Nursing Studies, MSc in Social Research, MA in Applied Professional Research) is a retired Senior Lecturer, who has taught in schools of nursing both in the West Midlands and the South East of England. She trained as a general nurse and a midwife and has varied general nursing experience. Just prior to her retirement, she returned to practice in a neuro-science centre as a lecturer-practitioner. This has further strengthened her belief that evidence-based practice in healthcare cannot be enforced without teaching professionals the skills to link research theory to practice. Her interest in teaching research and leading research modules over a period of 20 years have stemmed from her own Master's level studies, which have been in research methodologies. The challenge of ensuring methodological rigour while supervising undergraduate and postgraduate students with their literature review research projects convinced her of the need for this book. Her strong belief in a high standard of nurse education has led to her recent quality assurance role with the Nursing and Midwifery Council as an accredited reviewer of nursing programmes. This role is for six months of the year and the rest of her time is spent writing and enjoying her garden.

Dr Huguette Comerasamy (RN, RM, ADM, PGCEA, MSc (Ed Studies) PhD (Ed Studies) is a Principal Lecturer at the University of Brighton. Her speciality is midwifery and she teaches research across undergraduate and postgraduate levels in the Faculty of Health and Social Science. She has particular interests in the philosophical basis of research, literature-based research methodology and developing students as researchers. She believes that developing students as researchers ought to begin at an early stage in the curriculum. To this end, she has used the dissertation as a tool to engage undergraduate students with research. This has enabled students to develop research knowledge and skills that can serve as a platform for higher-order thinking about undertaking research in the future. She is the module leader for the dissertation module, which is based on literature review methodology, and she has taught research methodology for the past decade or so. She has also taught and conducted research seminars at the School of

Nursing in Mauritius, University of Iceland, University West Indies (St Augustine campus) and latterly University of Alberta, Canada. She is a member scholar of the International Institute of Qualitative Research, University of Alberta, Canada. Currently she supervises students' research projects at undergraduate and post-graduate levels and is an examiner of doctoral thesis both in the UK and abroad. Huguette is also a member of the editorial board of the *Journal of Obstetrics and Gynaecology* (UK).

Kate Clark (BLib, MCLIP) is Information Literacy Manager at the Royal College of Nursing where she has worked as part of the RCN's Library Archives and Information Services for 18 years. Her key role is to manage a programme of information literacy learning opportunities using face-to-face, web-conferencing technology and online methods. She works with members of the RCN, facilitating many learning opportunities herself. She has daily contact with the members, answering enquiries which frequently involve offering advice about sources of information and search strategies. Kate has worked with nurses for over 35 years. Having trained at the College of Librarianship Wales, University of Wales Aberystwyth, her first professional post was managing Normanby College Library, King's Health District (Teaching). Her work here included undertaking literatures searches for staff and teaching information literacy skills to student and qualified nurses, midwives, physiotherapists and radiographers. Her work at the RCN initially included undertaking literature searches, indexing journal articles for *Nursing Bibliography*, facilitating information literacy sessions and working with members in the Library and over the telephone. Recently, she has worked with RCN colleagues to develop and publish *Finding, Using and Managing Information: Nursing, Midwifery, Health and Social Care Information Literacy Competences* (Royal College of Nursing, 2011). She is passionate about helping nurses develop their information literacy competence, believing that the skills involved are essential in providing excellent evidence-based patient care. She is an honorary member of the King's College Hospital Nurses League. Kate has contributed to Chapter 4.

Dr Jacqueline Claudette Comerasamy (RN, RM, RNT/Dip Ed, BSc Health Studies, MSc Health Psychology, DBA (Doctor in Business and Administration) is Academic Head at Glyndwr University (London) and previously undergraduate Programme Director at the University of Glasgow. Formally trained in clinical nursing and nursing education, she has spent two decades practising in acute and long-term patient care environments, developing and implementing curriculum, managing undergraduate programmes and research projects. Her research scholarship is partially informed by her strong belief in students' need to have a firm grounding in research from the onset of their nursing and midwifery studies. She has taught research at both undergraduate and postgraduate levels and supervised students' research projects in the field of clinical nursing and nursing education, as well as supervising research projects with allied health professions. She has a particular interest in action research and has successfully co-ordinated a collaborative action research project on the evaluation of student experiences in a multidisciplinary healthcare environment. She was also the Deputy Director of HealthQwest Graduate School in 2009 (a consortium of research for West Scotland) where she organized the school research conference. At national and international conferences, she has disseminated her findings of several pieces of research work. Jacqueline has contributed to Chapter 5.

Preface

This book introduces a new research perspective on literature-based methodology called the comprehensive literature review. As a methodology, comprehensive literature review is about analyzing and synthesizing literature from both empirical and non-empirical sources, utilizing logical stages of the research process. It focuses on both deductive and inductive processes of problem solving.

The concept of this book evolved five years ago when we recognized that there was very little guidance on how to conduct a research project using pluralistic sources of literature as data. The book is a culmination of our experiences of teaching research and supervising students undertaking a literature-based research project. The ideas expressed in the book have been piloted with undergraduate and postgraduate students. From the pilots, the students have demonstrated abilities to design their comprehensive literature review as a distinct methodology in its own right.

Literature-based methodology for undergraduate and postgraduate students in nursing and midwifery is gaining popularity as a means of completing their research projects. Empirical research is becoming the reserve of those undertaking higher degrees, or who are qualified researchers, as ethical governance and time constraint precludes students from embarking on empirical research. This book provides an alternative methodology for students learning to undertake research as part of their degree.

As the title suggests, it is a basic text that guides students through their research projects. It is written for undergraduate and postgraduate students with familiarity of research knowledge. Although aimed at nursing and midwifery students, the principles of the comprehensive literature review methodology can be adopted across other disciplines and professions. This book is more than a text on research methodology; it is also about developing students as researchers to build research capacity. We firmly believe that this starts at undergraduate and postgraduate levels. The skills gained thereafter can be translated to higher levels of studies in future career development.

How to use this book

This book is a tool-kit for research project construction. Each chapter consists of a set of objectives outlining the goals that students need to achieve. There are student examples and student activities highlighted in boxes. The student examples are aimed at conceptualizing some of the abstract research theories by linking these to contemporary practice. The student activities complement the examples as they develop students' understanding of research. Simple answers to the activities are not provided as the intention is to nurture skills in problem solving, such as critical thinking and logical reasoning, to arrive at answers both individually and in a group.

There are visual representations in the form of figures, flowcharts and tables that complement the theoretical discussions in the text. All chapters conclude with end-of-chapter learning points. These are useful in evaluating students' own learning and in helping the students write their reflective accounts. Other than being useful for students, this book may also be a valuable resource for teachers of research and dissertation supervision.

Acknowledgements

There are a number of people who have helped us to make this book possible, but too many to name individually. However, we would like to thank the following people for their part in enabling us to complete this book.

We owe a special debt of gratitude to Dr Tom Lewis for believing in us and for providing constant moral support throughout the journey of writing. His critical eye and challenging discussion has been invaluable in confirming our ideas for this book. He has enthused us to delve deeper into the theoretical underpinning of literature review methodology.

We are indebted to our respective families for their unfailing support and understanding, especially when the journey proved difficult. A special thank you to John Bere for his willingness to proof-read the manuscript at first-hand, and for the numerous cups of tea to keep us invigorated. To Ann Hopkins, who provided professional assistance in proof-reading our material, we are grateful.

We would also like to thank Lesley Dowding as she was there at the outset of the planning of the book. Her sound advice was realistic and encouraging, and fuelled our motivation to achieve our goal.

Finally, we must express our thanks to the contributors, who worked untiringly to meet our targets. Their expertise on the subject matter added immensely to their relevant chapters and provided a conduit for the entire book.

ONE

Introduction to Research Concepts and Terminologies

┌─ **Aim and objectives** ─┐

The aim of this chapter is to introduce important research concepts and terminologies. By the end of the chapter you will be able to:

- Understand why research is important
- Understand the differences between qualitative and quantitative research
- Differentiate between non-empirical versus empirical research
- Appreciate the role of literature review methodology in non-empirical research
- Outline the steps in the research process for a project using the literature review methodology.

1.1 Introduction

Research in nursing and midwifery is relatively 'young' compared to other disciplines, such as medicine. Nurses and midwives have trod a stony path in the process of professionalization, but we have come a long way in embracing the arts and science duality of our profession. Nurses and midwives have the skill, knowledge and self-awareness to maintain the high standards of our work. These high standards can only be achieved through the use of evidence-based practice. In order to continue to reap the rewards of our accomplishment, nurses and midwives need to understand the importance of research.

Formal research has always been carried out by researchers, but it has been advocated that students in nursing and midwifery need to carry out research projects as part of their curriculum. Before embarking on their research projects, it is vital that students begin by examining the following three themes:

- The meaning of research
- Sources of knowledge
- The purpose of research.

The rest of this section will be devoted to an exploration of these themes. There will be student activities interspersed within the text. For those activities that require you to read and reflect on passages extracted from journals, we would suggest that you use a reflective framework that you are familiar with, such as Gibbs' (1988), Johns' (2004), Kolb's (1984), Schön's (1991) and Bradbury-Jones et al.'s (2009) reflective models.

1.1.1 The meaning of the word 'research'

In most academic texts, research is defined as an empirical inquiry, which needs to be conducted in a systematic and logical manner (Burns and Grove, 2003; Parahoo, 2006). However, the word 're-search' also implies revisiting or re-examining a topic of interest. The ultimate aim of research is to add to the body of knowledge about a topic. It has a cumulative effect; as more research is done, the greater is that body of knowledge on that or any topic. As a student, you can play an important role in this cumulative process of generating knowledge from research.

Knowledge from a philosophical standpoint is about a person's journey to gain familiarity, awareness or understanding of a subject through study or experience. The converse of this is the lack of knowledge and the impoverishment of insight that can lead to stupidity and selfishness (Grayling, 2002). This school of thought emphasizes an individual's need to perceive and discover so as to learn. We would like to involve you, the student, in this journey of discovery and perception. However, a lot of students we have met find that the start of this journey is made problematical by their misunderstanding of what research really is. It is therefore important to clarify some of these misunderstandings, as the subject of research is replete with jargon.

STUDENT ACTIVITY 1.1

Brainstorm the word 'research' and produce a mind-map. If you are not familiar with mind-maps, we would suggest that you refer to Tony Buzan at www.buzanworld.com/Mind_Maps.htm and see Buzan (2002).

Keep this mind-map because you will be referring to it in this chapter.

1.1.2 Sources of knowledge

The aim of research is to generate knowledge and we have defined knowledge as being gained from *study* and *experience*. In nursing and midwifery, knowledge is traditionally regarded as scientific knowledge, i.e. it is reliable and unchallenged (Chalmers, 2004). However, more recent thinking suggests that practice-based nursing/midwifery research is 'an art' (Morse, 1994; Denzin and Lincoln, 2005) because the creative work of practitioners generates research that is in search of both knowledge and truth. However, knowledge and truth are tentative as these concepts are both value- and culture-laden (Crotty, 2003). Therefore, there needs to be a differentiation between knowledge that is 'general' and that which is 'particular', in order to understand what is true and how it is gained.

STUDENT ACTIVITY 1.2

Please read the extract below from Oberle and Allen (2001: 148):

> In attempting to define 'advanced practice', we argue that nursing as such is teleological or goal directed with those goals being defined by the patient or client in interaction with the nurse. In helping the patient meet identified goals, the nurse requires two kinds of knowledge – general and particular. General includes theory (know why), pattern recognition (know what), and practical knowledge (know how). Particular (know who) is personal knowledge about the patient. The advanced practice nurse, by virtue of graduate education, is able to move beyond the familiar and experientially learned. He or she makes a deliberate attempt to situate self in dialectic between general and particular knowledge in such a way that the interplay opens possibilities. Knowing when a particular action would be most helpful is defined as practical wisdom. We argue that a highly developed sense of practical wisdom is the hallmark of advanced practice.

Now reflect on your own practice, taking note of the following:
Think of an advanced-level nurse or midwife you have worked with in the past who has helped a female client achieve her goal by knowing what, how and why about that client in addition to being aware of her own (i.e. the nurse's or midwife's) values, beliefs and culture.

- Is this advanced-level nurse or midwife utilizing her knowledge of the client's signs and symptoms to come to a diagnosis?
- Is she utilizing her social skills of communication in gaining a rapport with the client and/or her family?
- Is she helping the client and/or family by providing adequate treatment, care and advice, which is value-free and accepting of the client's choice?

In the example above, the advanced-level nurse or midwife used a combination of general and particular knowledge. General knowledge is the understanding of

---

what, how and why, acquired through education. The ultimate goal is the formulation of that general knowledge into concepts and theories; this is where research findings play an important role as a cornerstone of theory building.

Particular knowledge, on the other hand, is the understanding of self. This self-awareness is gained from being in touch with oneself, so as to be in touch with others. The move from general to particular knowledge requires experience, as the student learns from observations made in the real world. The process of making sense of one's experience occurs through reflection. Reflective practice is something that has been considered by many authors, such as Boud, Keogh and Walker (1985), Gibbs (1988), Schön (1991) and Johns (2004), and it provides the vital link between theory and practice.

To complete the discussion of sources of knowledge, one must appreciate that general knowledge and particular knowledge are on either end of a continuum. Figure 1.1 highlights the crucial position of research in the generation of knowledge in practice-based professions. The message we want to get across to you is that research forms the foundation on which future knowledge is based.

1.1.3 Purpose of research

Research generates knowledge and ultimately theory. However, there is good and bad research and in Chapter 5 we will be revisiting the process of critiquing research. This is a valuable skill that is part of the process of literature review research methodology. From now on, our discussion of research relates to 'good' or worthwhile research.

The purpose of research can be broadly put into these two categories. It can be used to:

- solve a problem; and/or
- illuminate a topic.

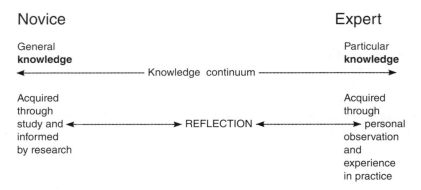

Figure 1.1 Knowledge continuum

Referring back to your mind-map of the meaning of research in Student Activity 1.1, can you see if your idea of research related to either of the above categories?

In our experience of facilitating students in their research, some have felt 'frustrated' as their chosen topic and process of research did not provide an immediate answer or a solution to the problem. This is not uncommon; it is human nature to seek spontaneous gratification. However, it is important to remember what we said earlier about knowledge being cumulative. If several pieces of research provide multiple perspectives on a problem, the total effect of illumination on a topic will ultimately point to an answer or a solution. This answer or solution may be the evidence needed to solve the problem and to justify action.

'Evidence-based healthcare' is a term that has been used more frequently in the last decade or so in the UK, and it is the backbone of quality assurance. Research is an irrefutable source of evidence to justify healthcare delivery (Brown, 2009). As practitioners, educationalists, managers and researchers, we need to be able to provide a rationale for our decisions and the actions we take. The consumers are our main stakeholders, but the benefits of our decisions and actions can be more far-reaching.

━━━━━━━━━━━━━━ **STUDENT ACTIVITY 1.4** ━━━━━━━━━━━━━━

Read the following four scenarios and determine the *stakeholders* concerned:

1 A podiatrist treated a diabetic foot with a new dressing used as part of a clinical trial devised by a pharmaceutical company.
2 A group of nurse teachers utilized a recently published method of visual collage with students to help develop reflective practice.
3 The director of public services based his decision on allocating funds to the development of a screening tool for domestic violence by referring to research done by a joint team of social workers and representatives from a crime prevention agency.
4 Two researchers from opposite sides of the world published their work on gene therapy in a well-known journal.

Discuss and compare your findings with another student. We hope you have come to the conclusion that the knock-on effect of evidence-based research can be far greater than you may have imagined.

n the above exercise, it is also interesting to note how evidence derived
research can be used to inform practice. The National Institute for Health
and Clinical Excellence (NICE) has, since April 1999, provided research-based
evidence for healthcare practitioners. These guidelines are developed for the
UK National Health Service in areas of public health, health technologies and
clinical practice. They are available for downloading from the website: www.
nice.org.uk.

The next section will explore the contrasting ways of thinking about research.
There are two traditional schools of thought on research, namely qualitative
and quantitative, but recent writings have indicated that an eclectic mix of
the two paradigms can be the way forward for contemporary research. Before
you delve into research using a mixed paradigm or mixed methodology, you
need to have a clear understanding of each of these two ways of thinking on
research.

1.2 Qualitative and quantitative: the contrasting paradigm

The polarization of research into the two contrasting schools brings us back
to our earlier discussion of problem solving. The qualitative research approach
looks at a problem or an issue from a different perspective than does quantitative
research. These epistemological perspectives or ways of thinking through a
problem or an issue are called paradigms.

Qualitative research or interpretivism is a way to gain insights through discovering meanings by improving our comprehension of the whole (Denzin
and Lincoln, 2005). The inductive paradigm, which is depicted in qualitative
research, is based on a humanistic view and a holistic philosophy, where the
emphasis is on the whole rather than its constituent parts.

Quantitative research or positivism utilizes scientific methods to uncover the
processes by which both physical and human events occur (Bowling, 2009).
The deductive paradigm, which is depicted in quantitative research, is based on
a reductionistic philosophy. This approach reduces a complex behaviour to a
simple set of variables that offer the possibility of identifying a cause-and-effect
relationship.

This section will concentrate on unpicking these two contrasting paradigms. It
will hopefully help you get a better understanding of why researchers favour one
of these ways of thinking over the other. Further discussion of the philosophical
basis of quantitative research (positivism) and qualitative research (interpretivism) is provided in Chapter 2.

1.2.1 Qualitative or inductive paradigm

Qualitative research epitomizes that which is meaningful and rich. In health-care, qualitative research focuses on abstract concepts, such as feelings, per-ceptions, experiences and to a certain extent attitudes, values and beliefs. The richness of the data collected is achieved through in-depth exploration of com-plex phenomena.

The qualitative researcher is constantly questioning the data presented to her/him, as the fluidity of the concept being explored challenges the researcher to frame and capture its meaning. Interpretation of the present-ing data is inevitable as the researcher attempts to make sense of the world of the researched (the participants). All this is what qualitative researchers aim to achieve as part of the process of theory construction. In other words, it is the mosaic composition of theory, piecing together snap-shots of data from the participants to create a whole picture. Qualitative researchers have long defended their paradigm as being rigorous and 'scientific'. They claim that all research (both qualitative and quantitative) involves judgement made by human minds by reference to human criteria. Human beings, especially researchers, are not computerized robots; their judgement cannot be totally objective. In order to be successful, qualitative researchers need to keep a check on their subjective influences.

Student Example 1.1   Qualitative paradigm

The following example presents an ex-student who has decided to utilize the quali-tative paradigm in his research:

James is a senior nurse at a colo-rectal unit. He is embarking on his postgraduate research project and wants to study changes in body image in patients who have had a stoma. Through prolonged interaction with stoma patients, James under-stands the *psychological impact* of such surgeries on patients and their families. He wants to discover the experience of these patients' 'psychological' journeys from diagnosis through to peri-operative and recovery periods.

James designs his research using the qualitative paradigm by *keeping an open mind on what he is discovering*. He collects data from talking to both stoma patients and their families about their experiences. By going through the processes of qualitative inquiry, James obtains a *wealth of data*, some of which confirms his understanding of what his patients and families are going through. There are also new findings that James uses to conceptualize mean-ing. All in all, the *construction of theory* in this inductive process provides James with a better understanding of how nurses can help in the care of these stoma patients.

From the above student example, you can take note of the essence of the *inductive paradigm in qualitative research*. It comprises:

- Exploring an abstract concept, such as psychological impact
- Discovering new meaning based on some pre-empted understanding, while keeping an open mind regarding the inductive process
- Obtaining a rich source of data from a small sample; some data confirm the paradigm whereas other evidence refutes it
- Constructing a theory as new meaning of the topic is conceptualized.

1.2.2 Quantitative or deductive paradigm

Quantitative research follows a strict set of rules to uncover complex phenomena. These rules are based on laws and predictions which are used to reach a conclusion from something that is already known (or assumed). The strength of quantitative research lies in its ability to utilize the process of inference or deduction so that human parameters, such as vital signs and other outcome measures, can be explained by simple principles of basic sciences.

Working in a different way from qualitative researchers, quantitative researchers set out to prove or refute a predicted outcome. The researcher needs to know all there is to know about the topic of exploration at the onset of the research so that all variables are taken into consideration. A theory or a set of theories are decided at the onset and subsequently tested by examining the relationships between the predetermined variables. In cases where no relationship between variables is found, the theory is simply described.

Student Example 1.2   Quantitative paradigm

The following example presents a student who has decided to utilize the quantitative paradigm in her research:

Yvonne is a third-year undergraduate student undertaking her research project as part of her midwifery course. She has just completed her placement on a labour ward where she witnessed different *outcomes* depending upon the way women were positioned in labour. Yvonne has a theory in mind and she wants to compare two different positions used in labour for primigravid women against the effects these have on the women's perineal health.

Yvonne designs her research project using the quantitative paradigm as she *already has a good idea of the problem* she wants to investigate. She selects her sample carefully by having a clear set of criteria. Data are collected from women's labour records. The *cause-and-effect relationship* is established between the two positions used in labour and the women's perineal health. *Large amounts of statistical data* are generated and the data are subsequently analyzed using a computer. By *excluding all other influencing variables*, Yvonne is able to come to a conclusion as to the *truthfulness of the theory* she set out to prove.

From the above student example, you can take note of the essence of the *deductive paradigm in quantitative research*. It comprises:

- Investigating a concrete concept, such as effect on outcomes
- Proving or disproving a problem or a hypothesis for which the investigator already has a pre-set idea as to its possible outcome(s)
- Obtaining statistical data from a large sample
- Focusing on the cause-and-effect relationship by excluding influencing factors
- Theory testing by confirming or refuting the truthfulness of existing theory

So far in this section on paradigms, we have looked at how either a qualitative paradigm or a quantitative paradigm can be utilized in nursing and midwifery research as pure entities. The following section will examine ways of mixing these in the design of research.

1.2.3 Mixed methodologies

The terms 'methodology' and 'methods' are not synonymous and they need to be clearly differentiated. Crotty (2003: 3) provides the following definitions:

> Methodology is the strategy, plan of action, process or design lying behind the choice and use of particular methods and linking the choice and use of methods to the desired outcomes.
>
> Methods are the techniques and procedures used to gather and analyse data related to some research question or hypothesis.

Tashakkori and Teddlie (2003) use the term 'mixed methods research' to refer to all procedures for collecting and analyzing quantitative and qualitative data in the context of a single study. The triangulation of these various procedures or processes in a single study further reinforces research rigour. Discussion of the use of triangulation to boost rigour in research using mixed methods will be elaborated in Chapter 7.

Research using mixed methodologies stems from the differing perspectives on problem solving: one using inductive reasoning (qualitative) and the other using deductive reasoning (quantitative). These two logical ways of solving problems are both workable; qualitative research and quantitative research can stand alone in their own right as 'pure' methodologies. This was illustrated in the student examples in the previous section. However, in the last decade or so, research utilizing both paradigms has become more common. This mixed methodology values the strengths of both qualitative and quantitative research (Depoy and Gitlin, 2005).

The following sections provide examples of how the two contrasting paradigms can be used in problem solving/logical reasoning by the formation of sequential loops.

1.2.3.1 The qualitative–quantitative loop

Figure 1.2 illustrates the use of mixed methodology in the *theory construction – testing loop*. The initial inductive reasoning process in a qualitative design contributes to the construction of a preliminary theory, which can be tested using a quantitative design on a larger sample of the target population. This will allow confirmation of the initial theory; and with the subsequent generation of new theory, the qualitative–quantitative loop of research will be further reiterated.

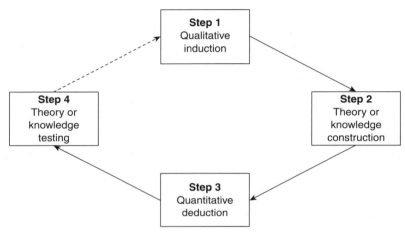

Figure 1.2   Qualitative–quantitative loop

Student Example 1.3   Mixed methodology using the qualitative–quantitative loop

In healthcare research, qualitative evidence has been used as a precursor to quantitative research, such as facilitating questionnaire design or in determining the selection of an outcome measure. The abstract below has been taken from published research that illustrates the use of qualitative followed by quantitative mixed methodology:

> In this article, the authors demonstrate how qualitative methods can form a foundation for quantitative research by improving instrument validity, informing the data collection process, and improving cost-effectiveness in a study of physician decision-making. To test terminology, applicability, and comprehension of a quantitative questionnaire for doctors in the United States and United Kingdom, each country's researchers conducted physician focus groups with questions organized around the experiment, including (a) validity of video vignettes of actor 'patients', (b) population accessibility, (c) level of remuneration, (d) appropriate endorsement figure, and (e) question comprehension. Focus group data collected during instrument development and fieldwork planning streamlined processes and achieved cost efficiencies and effectiveness for

the overall study. Beyond simply adding a post hoc qualitative component to an already freestanding quantitative methodology, focus groups were used in the study formulation, where the qualitative methodology was integrated into the process of developing a valid survey instrument. (O'Donnell et al., 2007: 971)

Discuss with another student the usefulness of the above research by examining some of the following points:

- Conducting discussions with a pre-selected group of doctors prior to the development of a questionnaire.
- Watching a video of actor 'patients' to get the doctors to think through how they make decisions themselves.
- Questioning the ethics behind the use of remunerations or 'inducements' to recruit doctors for the quantitative survey.

We hope you find in your discussion that the preliminary work, in the form of qualitative research, was necessary and vital in strengthening the use of questionnaires for the survey design in the next stage of the research.

1.2.3.2 The quantitative–qualitative loop

Figure 1.3 illustrates the use of mixed methodology in a *theory testing–construction loop*. This time the initial deductive reasoning process in a quantitative design allows testing of an existing theory on a larger sample of the population. This is followed by further exploration of a selected small sample, either as a subset of the original sample or from a new sample. This subsequent inductive process will generate new knowledge, which may support or attenuate the original theory tested in the deductive process.

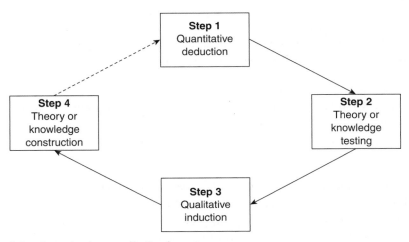

Figure 1.3   Quantitative–qualitative loop

Student Example 1.4 Mixed methodology using the quantitative–qualitative loop

Quantitative numeric techniques used in the initial stage of the research are predominantly descriptive. This is followed by the qualitative explanatory phase, which helps to explore outlier cases emerging from the descriptive phase. The abstract below has been taken from a published research that illustrates the use of quantitative followed by qualitative mixed methodology:

> Personal digital assistants (PDAs) are increasingly in use in both clinical practice and nursing education as a method of providing timely access to resources at the point of care. This article describes the use of PDAs during the medical-surgical clinical component of a Bachelor of Nursing program in Australia. The aim of the study was to investigate whether PDAs would enhance students' pharmacological and clinical contextual knowledge and to identify issues associated with the use of PDAs in students' clinical experience. A mixed-method approach was used incorporating a quasi-experimental design with pre-test and post-test of pharmacological knowledge and focus group discussions. Students using the PDAs demonstrated a moderate increase in their mean score, which was double the increase in the control group. Findings from the focus group discussions indicated that students found the PDAs easy to use and perceived their use as beneficial to their learning in the clinical area. This study provides support for the ongoing implementation of PDAs into nursing education. (Farrell and Rose, 2008: 13)

Discuss with another student the usefulness of the above research by examining some of the following points:

- Gathering students' perceptions of the use of mobile handheld computers or PDAs in clinical practice in a focus group discussion
- Testing the students' pharmacological knowledge before and after using the PDAs in clinical practice
- Qualitative comments from the students indicated that the computers were easy to use and that the computers did actually benefit their learning.

We hope you find in your discussion that the follow-up qualitative research not only helped to reinforce the findings, but was useful in exploring the reasons for this particular outcome of the initial quasi-experiment.

So far we have talked about a *sequential* approach to mixed methodology research, with the possibilities of completing the paradigm loop. However, several writers have also highlighted the *concurrent* approach to mixed methodology research (Tashakkori and Teddlie, 2003; Flemming, 2007; Andrew and Halcomb, 2009).

This has been likened to the spiral of the DNA double helix (Mendlinger and Cwikel, 2008). However, a word of caution is needed. Research using the mixed methodological design is time-consuming as it involves careful planning and a sound knowledge of the paradigms. In this book, the proposed methodology of comprehensive literature review utilizes a mixed methodology in both sequential and concurrent approaches. This will be elaborated in subsequent chapters.

The next section will begin with the introduction of more research terms. It is important that you understand these as they form the basis of the backbone of this book, which is the need to design a literature review methodology in parallel with empirical research.

1.3 Empirical and non-empirical research

At the start of this section, it is important for you to differentiate between empirical and non-empirical research. In empirical research, the researcher uses a logical stepwise approach to pursue knowledge. By virtue of the researcher being immersed in the real world, *primary data* is collected from the sample population through this step-by-step process.

On the other side of the coin, although the term 'non-empirical' is quoted in a spectrum of professional literature, ranging from educational, business through to social science and health, the word 'non-empiricism' basically refers to anything that is not observed or experienced in the real world. Non-empirical research is the gathering of *secondary sources of data* taken from the findings of primary research.

The *Journal of Interdisciplinary Health Sciences* (www.hsag.co.za 2010) provides clear guidelines for authors submitting non-empirical research to their journal. They define four types of non-empirical research (see Table 1.1):

- Philosophical analysis
- Literature review
- Conceptual analysis
- Theory or model building.

Of the four types of non-empirical research typology described in Table 1.1, the *literature review methodology* is the most appropriate and valuable type of research for undergraduate and postgraduate students in health and social care.

1.3.1 The value of non-empirical research

There is no doubt that the turn of the century has heralded a technological explosion. Information is now accessible in a quantity and at a speed beyond the imagination of our forefathers. Personal data are no longer the premise of

Table 1.1 The four types of non-empirical research

Philosophical analysis	Literature review	Conceptual analysis	Theory or model building
The literature analysis for the philosophical analysis aims at analyzing arguments or debates in favour of or against a particular position. One can distinguish, e.g. normative analysis, ideology critique, phenomenological analysis or deconstruction applications of philosophical analysis.	*A comprehensive and a critical analysis of the literature should be provided that illustrates the different theoretical perspectives, trends or debates with regard to the phenomenon under investigation. The literature review should be presented in a clear, comprehensive and balanced (objective) way. The literature analysis should reflect a high quality of scientific argumentation and logic in the identification of the limitations/ deficiencies in existing theory/methodology. The arguments around these deficiencies/limitations should be presented in a coherent and systematic manner. Existing theoretical perspectives on these problems/issues should be fully and clearly presented.*	The literature analysis for conceptual analysis should be characterized by clarification and elaboration of the meaning of words and concepts through either generic differentiation or conditional type of conceptual analysis.	In the case of theory or model building, the literature study will be characterized by a search for linkages between theoretical ideas or concepts in order to find coherence, an explanation for or a causal link between theoretical propositions. It is aimed at explaining phenomena through a new theory, hypothesis or model.

private individuals. Data generated from research have multiplied to such an extent that what is in the public domain needs to be protected. The government has therefore legislated to protect the general public from researchers. This is in the form of the Data Protection Act (UK Legislation 1998), the Freedom of Information Act (UK Legislation 2000) and arguably the most important publication in 2001, the *Research Governance Framework for Health and Social Care* (DOH, 2001). The responsibilities of individuals such as the participants, researchers, research sponsors and organizations (universities and care providers alike) are clearly stated in this framework document. Since its publication, universities have responded by producing their own research guidelines. Undergraduate students in health and social care settings are no longer allowed to undertake empirical research. Postgraduate students in these same settings are closely monitored by their supervisors, and strict regulations need to be adhered to when submitting research proposals to ethics committees and academic gatekeepers who are people/authorities that hold the power to sanction data collection from patients, healthcare staff and co-students.

Although one can understand the need for caution as vulnerable individuals can easily be exploited, this situation means that undergraduate students in health and social care settings are not embarking on any research. The effect has been to stifle their research enthusiasm and skill development. Since undergraduate students are required to submit a research project as part of their degree, non-empirical research has come to play an increasingly important part, particularly that of the literature review methodology. Nurse and midwife researchers have saturated the research arena with findings that require closer review. Thus the use of literature review as a methodology for student research projects satisfies two important needs: that of rigorous scrutiny of findings produced by nurse and midwife researchers and the opportunity for these students to understand and put into practice the research process.

1.3.2 What is literature review methodology?

We cannot emphasize enough that *literature review* is a research methodology. It is important to carry out this non-empirical research in a rigorous manner by incorporating all the stages of the research process. It is a research methodology in which the choice of research method is the review of published research and their findings. The methodology, therefore, is the strategy, plan of action, process or design lying behind the choice and use of this literature review method (Crotty, 2003).

The research design advocated in this book is *comprehensive*. A range of research literature from a pluralistic source is sampled, reviewed, critiqued, analyzed and interpreted. This follows a rigorous process, which is a required component of any sound methodology. The wide range of research literature can be either qualitative or quantitative research or a mix of the two methodologies.[1] Gorard (2002) challenges entrenched views about the relationship between qualitative and quantitative research being opposing views of the theoretical underpinning of research. He suggests that the way forward is to avoid allegiances to either methodology and to recognize that no methodology is preferable to any other. The choice of methodology should be based on fitness for purpose, i.e. will it answer the question that the research seeks to answer? To do so, you will need to follow the chosen 'route' of problem solving through its rightful research processes. These research processes are elaborated in the next section of this chapter.

1.4 The research process

The last section of this chapter provides a summary of what has been discussed so far. The stages of the research process will set the scene for the remaining chapters in this book. When defining the research process, Parahoo (2006) claims that research starts with questions raised from reflective practice. The systematic and rigorous stages which follow include data collection and analysis, and these must be communicated transparently for all to see in the form of oral and/or written presentations.

Although the actual stages of the research process are generic, there are still differences between empirical and non-empirical research. Literature review methodology as a type of non-empirical research, utilizes a slightly different research process, because secondary sources of data (as opposed to primary research) are the mainstay of the research itself.

1.4.1 Empirical research process and literature review methodology research process compared

In empirical research, the quantitative research process differs from that of the qualitative process. The quantitative research process tends to follow a linear pattern, whereby one process is completed before the next. Qualitative research, on the other hand, is less regimental as the stages of the process (especially those of data collection and analysis) tend to be iterative and can be described as cyclical (Polit and Beck, 2010).

In the literature review methodology, the process of research is dependent on the paradigmatic mindset of the researcher. From the start, you must be clear as to whether you are using an inductive or deductive reasoning process in problem solving as this will determine the later research stages. The research process for empirical and non-empirical research is summarized in Table 1.2. The literature review methodology differs from that of the empirical research process in just five out of the ten stages (highlighted bold in Table 1.2).

The ten stages of the research process listed in the right-hand column of Table 1.2 will form the subject matter of the remaining chapters of this book.

By way of summary, Table 1.3 compares qualitative and quantitative research and the stages of the research process in both empirical and non-empirical research.

Table 1.2 Comparison of the two types of research process

Empirical research process	Non-empirical (literature review methodology) research process
1. Identifying the research problem or topic	1. Identifying the research problem or topic
2. Deciding on the research question(s) or hypothesis(es) after a preliminary review of the literature	2. Deciding on the research question(s) or hypothesis(es) after a preliminary review of the literature
3. **Choosing the right research design (quantitative, qualitative or mixed methodology)**	3. **Choosing a comprehensive literature review by considering findings from qualitative/quantitative research and grey literature**
4. **Deciding on the sample**	4. **Deciding on the sample of literature based on the identified research problem or topic**
5. **Collecting data**	5. **Collecting data by searching the literature**
6. **Considering ethics for ethical clearance**	6. **Considering ethics when critiquing the literature**
7. **Analyzing data**	7. **Analyzing literature-based data**
8. Considering research rigour	8. Considering research rigour
9. Discussing and writing up the results	9. Discussing and writing up the results
10. Implementing and disseminating findings	10. Implementing and disseminating findings

End-of-Chapter Learning Points

We hope you have had time to reflect on what you have learnt from the student activities. The following are some of the key points highlighted in this chapter:

1 Knowledge is cumulative. We *all* play a part in contributing to the body of knowledge generated through research.
2 The benefits of research are multiple and this is underpinned by its purpose.
3 Qualitative and quantitative research complement each other and the eclectic approach of mixed methodologies strengthens the quality of the research findings generated.
4 Empirical research generates primary data or findings, which are subsequently used as a secondary source for non-empirical research.
5 Non-empirical research using the literature review methodology allows healthcare practitioners to reflect on and draw together primary research findings.

Table 1.3 Summary comparing qualitative and quantitative research and the stages of the research process in both empirical and non-empirical research

Research process	Empirical research		Non-empirical research (using literature review methodology)	
	Qualitative research	Quantitative research	Qualitative research	Quantitative research
1. Identifying the research problem/topic	• Abstract concept • Inductive reasoning: ending up with theory (theory construction) • Use of research questions	• Concrete concept • Deductive reasoning: theory up-front (theory testing) • Use of hypothesis(es) or aims and objectives	Same as empirical research (Chapter 2)	
2. Preliminary review of the literature	• Minimal at the onset	• Extensive	Same as empirical research (Chapter 2)	
3. Research design or approach	For example: • Phenomenology • Grounded theory • Ethnography	For example: • True experiments or randomized control trials • Quasi-experiments • Surveys	Comprehensive literature review methodology (Chapter 3)	
4. Deciding on the sample • Sampling process • Size of sample • Sample characteristics	For example: • Non-probability sampling (e.g. convenience sampling) • Small sample: 5–10 (approximately) • No or 'loose' inclusion and exclusion criteria	For example: • Probability sampling (e.g. random sampling) • Large sample: >100 • Clear inclusion and exclusion criteria	With clear inclusion and exclusion criteria in mind, findings from both qualitative and quantitative research are used as secondary sources of data (Chapter 4)	
5. Collecting data	For example: • Unstructured questionnaires • In-depth interviews • Participant observation	For example: • Structured questionnaires • Structured interviews • Non-participant observation	Searching and sampling the literature (Chapter 4)	

	Empirical research		Non-empirical research (using literature review methodology)	
Research process	Qualitative research	Quantitative research	Qualitative research	Quantitative research
6. Considering ethics: • Local research ethics committee clearance • Informed consent	Same for both: • Patient information sheet • Consent form	Same for both: • Patient information sheet • Consent form	Ethical considerations when critiquing the literature (Chapter 5)	
7. Analyzing data	For example: • Content or thematic analysis	For example: • Statistical analysis using computer • Descriptive statistics • Inferential statistics	Analysis of findings from qualitative/quantitative research and grey literature (Chapter 6)	
8. Considering research rigour	Four criteria of trustworthiness (Lincoln and Guba, 1985): • Credibility • Transferability • Dependability • Confirmability	Reliability and validity as the quantitative measure of rigour	Four ways of boosting rigour and awareness of ethical underpinnings (Chapter 5 and 7)	
9. Discussing and writing up results	• Results presented with quotes from transcripts or field notes • Findings supported by literature	• Results presented in diagrammatic format • Findings proves or disproves hypothesis(es)	Same as empirical research (Chapter 7 and 8)	
10. Implementing and disseminating findings	• Same in both	• Same in both	Same as empirical research	

Note

1 Please note that the discussion here is about research literature. Other sources of data, such as grey literature, will be mentioned in subsequent chapters of this book.

References

On reflection

Boud, D., Keogh, R. and Walker, D. (eds) (1985) *Reflection: Turning Experience into Learning*. New York: Routledge Falmer.

Bradbury-Jones, C., Hughes, S.M., Murphy, W., Parry, L. and Sutton, J. (2009) 'A new way of reflecting in nursing: the Peshkin Approach', *Journal of Advanced Nursing*, 65(11), 2485–2493.

Buzan, T. (2002) *How to Mind Map: The Thinking Tool That Will Change Your Mind*. London: Thorsons.

Gibbs, G. (1988) *Learning by Doing: A Guide to Teaching and Learning Methods*. Oxford: Further Education Unit, Oxford Polytechnic.

Johns, C. (2004) *Becoming a Reflective Practitioner* (2nd edn). Oxford: Blackwell.

Kolb, D.A. (1984) *Experiential Learning: Experience as a Source of Learning and Development*. Upper Saddle River, NJ: Prentice-Hall.

Schön, D.A. (1991) *The Reflective Practitioner: How Professionals Think in Action*. New York: Basic Books.

On evidence-based nursing

Brown, S.J. (2009) *Evidence-Based Nursing: The Research-Practice Connection*. Sudbury, MA: Jones and Bartlett.

Flemming, K. (2007) 'The knowledge base for evidence-based nursing: a role for mixed methods research?', *Advances in Nursing Science*, 30(1), 41–51.

On general nursing

Chalmers, A.F. (2004) *What is This Thing Called Science?* (3rd edn). Milton Keynes: Open University Press.

Grayling, A.C. (2002) *The Meaning of Things: Applying Philosophy to Life*. London: Phoenix.

Oberle, K. and Allen, M. (2001) 'The nature of advanced practice nursing', *Nursing Outlook*, 49(3), 148–153.

On general research

Bowling, A. (2009) *Research Methods in Health: Investigating Health and Health Services* (3rd edn). Maidstone: McGraw-Hill/Open University Press.

Burns, N. and Grove, S.K. (2003) *Understanding Nursing Research* (3rd edn). Philadelphia, PA: W.B. Saunders.

Crotty, M. (2003) *The Foundations of Social Research: Meaning and Perspective in Social Research*. London: Sage.

Denzin, N.K. and Lincoln, Y.S. (eds) (2005) *Handbook of Qualitative Research* (3rd edn). London: Sage.

Department of Health (2001) *Research Governance Framework for Health and Social Care*, Chapter 3. London: HMSO.

Depoy, E. and Gitlin, L.N. (2005) *Introduction to Research Understanding and Applying Multiple Strategies* (3rd edn). St Louis, MO: Mosby.

Morse, J.M. (ed.) (1994) *Critical Issues in Qualitative Research Methods*. Thousand Oats, CA: Sage.

Parahoo, K. (2006) *Nursing Research: Principles, Process and Issues* (2nd edn). Basingstoke: Palgrave Macmillan.

Polit, D.F. and Beck, C.T. (2010) *Essentials of Nursing Research: Appraising Evidence for Nursing Practice* (7th edn). Philadelphia, PA: Wolters Kulwer Health/Lippincott, Williams & Wilkins.

On general mixed methodology

Andrew, S. and Halcomb, E.J. (2009) *Mixed Methods Research for Nursing and the Health Sciences*. Chicester: Wiley-Blackwell.

Farrell, M.J. and Rose, L. (2008) 'Use of mobile handheld computers in clinical nursing education', *Journal of Nursing Education*, 47(1), 13–19.

Gorard, S. (2002) 'Can we overcome the methodological schism? Four models for combining qualitative and quantitative evidence', *Research Papers in Education*, 17(4), 345–361.

Mendlinger, S. and Cwikel, J. (2008) 'Spiraling between qualitative and quantitative data on women's health behaviors: a double helix model for mixed methods', *Qualitative Health Research*, 18(2), 280–293.

O'Donnell, A.B. et al. (2007) 'Using focus group to improve the validity of cross-national survey research: a study of physician decision making', *Qualitative Health Research,* 17(7), 971–981.

Tashakkori, A. and Teddlie, C. (eds) (2003) *Handbook of Mixed Methods in Social and Behavioural Research*. Thousand Oaks, CA: Sage.

UK Legislation (1998) *Data Protection Act*, Chapter 7. London: HMSO.

UK Legislation (2000) Freedom of Information Act, Chapter 1. London: HMSO.

Websites

On mind-maps: www.buzanworld.com/Mind_Maps.htm

Journal of Interdisciplinary Health Sciences Author Guidelines: www.hsag.co.za/index.php/HSAG/about/submissions.

TWO

Identifying the Research Problem

Aim and objectives

The aim of this chapter is to focus on the processes involved in, and the underpinning philosophical basis of, identifying a research problem. It then discusses how to use this knowledge to generate a research question or statement. By the end of this chapter you will be able to:

- Understand the different types of knowledge in relation to the historical and philosophical perspectives of research
- Understand the role of philosophical underpinning in supporting the choice of research methodology
- Appreciate the complexity of identifying a research problem
- Generate and refine a research question or statement.

2.1 Introduction

As you have seen in Chapter 1, research is about the generation of knowledge. In fact the creation and use of knowledge are the motivating forces behind research. Along with understanding the 'why' of research, you have also developed an understanding of the research methodology and the different approaches that may be used to generate new knowledge or new insights into knowledge.

When ascertaining how nursing and midwifery ought to develop knowledge using research approaches, it is vital that we begin by examining three main themes pertaining to knowledge:

- Scope of knowledge
- Ontological issues
- Epistemological issues.

Before exploring these themes, we present a conceptual framework developed by the authors (in Figure 2.1) to provide an overview of the scope of nursing and midwifery knowledge. The purpose is to contextualize the issues that are present in each of the three themes listed above. It will also lead us to consider areas that we might not otherwise explore.

Although the conceptual framework in Figure 2.1 suggests that nursing and midwifery knowledge come from different epistemic orientations, they share a unifying element, which is dealing with humankind. There is little doubt that the field of nursing and midwifery has a rich history of practice and with it a rich knowledge-base – knowledge that has yet to be validated by research. Suffice to say that the root of knowledge in both fields come from other disciplines, such as anthropology and sociology. Let us return to the very reason for research, which is the intent to create knowledge. First, then, we need to look

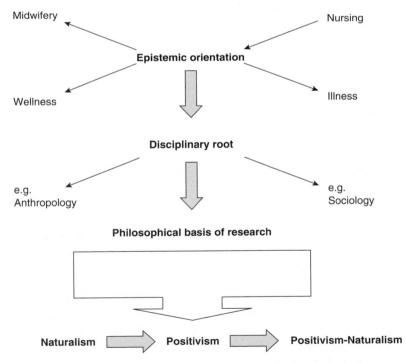

Figure 2.1   An overview of the scope of nursing and midwifery knowledge: a conceptual framework

at the types of knowledge, the ways of knowing, or even to ask ourselves what counts as knowledge?

You need to begin thinking about your research problem with the above in mind because during the process of designing a research project it is not unusual to come across some knowledge or ways of knowing that are unfamiliar but which are necessary to the problem you want to solve.

2.2 Defining the scope of knowledge

In this section we advance what has been covered in Chapter 1 (section 1.1.2) on the 'Sources of Knowledge'. In talking about the scope of knowledge, we refer to types of knowledge. Nursing and midwifery have rested mainly on medical knowledge, which has been generated through quantitative methodology, which claims to be scientific. It is no longer sufficient for nursing and midwifery to simply identify with medical knowledge. Rather, as nurses and midwives, we need to reacquaint ourselves with other types of knowledge that existed before the advent of modern medicine. Tables 2.1 and 2.2 show the types of knowledge discussed by other authors.

Table 2.1 Belief systems (Parahoo, 2006: 31)

1. Mythical or theological beliefs
2. Metaphysical beliefs
3. Scientific beliefs

Table 2.2 Ways of knowing (Burns and Grove, 2001: 12)

1. Traditions – based on past customs and trends. Bluett and Cluff (2000: 13) add: 'This is the way we have always done it'.

2. Authority – this is based on a person's expertise and power to influence opinion and behaviour.

3. Borrowing – from disciplines such as medicine, psychology, physiology, sociology.

4. Trial and error – used when there are no other sources of knowledge.

5. Personal experience – involves gaining knowledge by being involved in a situation or event. As more experience is gained, the person's repertoire of knowledge increases.

6. Role-modelling and mentorship – learning through interaction with or following the examples of the role-modeller/mentor.

The purpose of research, as you learnt in Chapter 1, is to generate knowledge. This is also done by building on existing knowledge. Now reflect on the following two scenarios:

Scenario 1

Having been diagnosed with colonic cancer, Jane is admitted to your ward for surgery. After she has settled in, you go to talk to her about the necessary preparation for surgery, which has been scheduled for the next day. You notice that she had a peacock feather on her locker. She is adamant about her decision to display it there. To her this is a symbol of trust.

Scenario 2

Some 20 years ago when she was just 3 years old, Affssa, a little girl originally from Somalia but now a migrant in the UK, was circumcised (a practice known to us as female genital mutilation or FGM). Affssa is 20 weeks pregnant when you first meet her at the antenatal clinic. Talking to her, you find that she is proud of who she has become. She is able to tell you about her attitudes regarding her body and the reason why she agrees with the cultural practice of FGM.

After reflecting on the above scenarios, examine the types of knowledge presented in Tables 2.1 and 2.2 and construct a mind-map.

- In the mind-map, include your *own knowledge* by comparing this to the conceptual framework of nursing and midwifery in Figure 2.1.
- Then include *the knowledge that the client* brings with them to the practice of nursing and midwifery.

Keep this mind-map as you will need it for later activities, particularly when you begin to identify your research problem.

From the above exercise, you will have noted that nursing and midwifery knowledge is not as straightforward as you might have envisaged. We bring with us our understanding of knowledge and, with it, our belief system about what counts as knowledge. In the next section, we will explore these factors in relation to nursing and midwifery research.

2.3 Philosophical underpinnings of research and their application to nursing and midwifery

The philosophical underpinnings of research are broad subjects; they cannot be addressed fully in this section and it is not our intention to do so. For the purpose of this section, we will look at two main issues upon which the choice of methodology rests. These are called ontology and epistemology.

Ontology and epistemology are two major aspects of a branch of philosophy called metaphysics (Guba, 1990). Often the terms ontology and epistemology are used interchangeably. While they are indeed connected, they differ in meaning and it is worth spending some time examining them in order to understand how they inform research methodology.

These terms are not always elaborated in published research, but they are of great significance when designing a research project and when critically evaluating work conducted by other researchers. There are three main reasons for understanding the philosophical underpinnings of research:

1 They provide a theoretical framework for understanding the assumptions we make about reality (Clough and Nutbrown, 2000).
2 They allow us to contextualize our research problem, formulate research questions/statements and justify our methodological approach.
3 They allow us to apply rigorous criteria when we are critically examining the stances of researchers and the rigour of published research findings.

2.3.1 Ontology

Ontology is a concept that refers to what is real. It asks the question: 'what is the nature of reality or what is the nature of the world?' (Guba, 1990: 18). This concept might be further developed by suggesting that ontology refers to people, contexts and belief systems which we might call the real world. Of course there is a real world out there, but what that real world is, and how it is defined and experienced is dependent upon our belief system or paradigm (Guba, 1990; Denzin and Lincoln, 1998). Given that the world is made up of different people, contexts and belief systems, it makes sense that there is more than one reality (often referred to as multi-realities), and thus these are different ways of experiencing and living that reality. As we have already mentioned, Parahoo (2006: 31) identifies three specific realities. These are: mythical or theological beliefs, metaphysical beliefs and scientific beliefs.

It is fair to say that there are many ways of knowing and that people bring with them ways of knowing from their reality, that is their culture, their educational background and possibly their beliefs and values. Imagine the field of nursing and midwifery as *professional worlds*, which are populated by a wide range of people. Examples of these people are nurses, doctors with different specialisms and midwives, and all offer services to clients in their *everyday life world*. Sometimes the professionals' ways of knowing may be incompatible with the nature of what is happening in the clients' everyday life world.

To summarize, our understanding of what constitutes reality is an equally important consideration in situating the research within the appropriate paradigm or school of thought. You need to be mindful that each individual comes from and experiences a different reality.

████████████████████ **STUDENT ACTIVITY 2.2** ████████████████████

Refer to your mind-map in Student Activity 2.1 and see if you can make the following connections:

- Which of the types of knowledge in your mind-map relate to people, contexts or belief systems?
- Of the belief systems, which of these belong to mythical or theological beliefs, meta-physical beliefs and scientific beliefs?
- In relation to the context or the ways of knowing about their world, which of these fall under the influence of culture, educational background and possibly beliefs and values?

Share your answers with another student and discuss the mind-maps you have constructed. Appreciate the fact that each of your mind-maps may be different, but try to arrive at an understanding as to why they are different.

2.3.1.1 The different types of ontology

The different ontologies that inform or are informed by nursing and midwifery research can therefore be classified as follows:

1 **Realist ontology** (Guba, 1990) – is the belief that reality exists out there but that it is one that is driven by natural laws. The aim of research in this context is to discover the true nature of that reality and find out how it works. As you have learnt in Chapter 1, the purpose of deductivistic research is to predict and control phenomena (refer to Figure 2.3 when discussing quantitative methodology).
2 **Relativist ontology** (Guba, 1990) – realities are seen to exist in the form of multiple mental constructions, socially and experientially based, local and specific, depending on their form and content on the persons who hold them. In other words, as Willis (2007: 48) claims, 'the reality we perceive is always conditioned by our experiences', which is the purpose of inductivistic research (refer to Figure 2.4 when discussing qualitative methodology).

This indicates that there are different starting points or positions to be taken into account when seeking to generate knowledge. These are referred to as philosophical positions. Let us stretch this idea further and relate it to nursing and midwifery practice by referring to Figure 2.2 and then completing Student Activity 2.3.

Medical staff, nurses, midwives and of course clients will have varying belief systems and all will be influenced by the different contexts. This is illustrated in Figure 2.2.

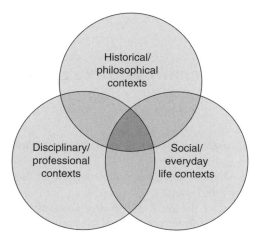

Figure 2.2 The contexts of belief systems (adapted from Paterson et al., 2001)

Ask a client how he/she perceives the situation that he/she is in. Choose from either of the following:

1 Ask a pregnant woman what she knows about pregnancy. Now compare these findings with what you have learnt from textbook knowledge or other sources.
2 Ask a client suffering from diabetes what he/she knows about the condition and compare these findings with what you have learnt from textbook knowledge or other sources.

Now share your findings of the similarities and differences with another student and discuss the following points:

• What are the factors that influence your understanding and perception of the situation?
• Try to group these factors under the three contexts illustrated in Figure 2.2.

2.3.2 Epistemology

Epistemology is another philosophical concept which may be regarded as the twin concept of ontology. It is about the theory of knowledge and is essentially asking 'how do we know what we know?' (Guba, 1990; Clough and Nutbrown, 2000; Willis, 2007). Epistemology is the path to knowledge construction and in research terms this is what is referred to as methodology (Guba, 1990: 18).

Establishing knowledge is a complex process involving our belief systems. It is based on different schools of thought with contrasting paradigms and evolved within the Enlightenment movement of the seventeenth century. Science was considered to be the supreme form of knowledge since this knowledge was created by means of observation and experimentation. This is the key characteristic of scientific (quantitative) methodology and differentiates it from metaphysical and religious knowledge (Chalmers, 1990). According to Descartes (1968/1637), scientific (quantitative) methodology is the key to expanding all human knowledge. It is the origin of the philosophical basis of research methodology known as the positivist school of thought.

2.3.2.1 The positivist school of thought

The positivists believe that there is one single objective reality about the world. It provides the theoretical basis of all quantitative research. The major influence is Descartes (1968/1637), who envisaged scientific methodology as the key to expanding all knowledge, thus enabling human beings to gain control over knowledge expansion. Looking back at the historical development of nursing and midwifery, you will recognize the contribution of knowledge that the positivist has made to both disciplines. Descartes (1968/1637) extolled the notions of objectivity, subjectivity and value-neutrality, which became the dominant values in science (quantitative research). An example of objectivity and value-neutrality, as most research texts will attest, is simply that the researcher is not involved with those being researched. By being detached from those being researched, researchers, in effect, hold no bias and are value-free. We can argue that this is indeed so because the researcher sees that data are in isolation from the person from whom the data was obtained. The following example illustrates this point.

Student Example 2.1   Positivism

Remember Yvonne, the student midwife in Chapter 1? She was interested in conducting an experiment on the relationship between labour positions and outcome in the form of women's perineal health. Yvonne was using the women's labour records to extract data. This method of research depended on observations made by other midwife colleagues. By collecting data in this fashion, she detached herself from the clients, who were the women themselves.

This example underlines the essence of positivism, as the researcher (Yvonne) is not biased by the women's presentation or description of their labour outcomes.

To sum up, the specific research methodology deriving from the positivist school of thought is the quantitative methodology discussed in Chapter 1. As you have learned there, the reasoning explicit in quantitative methodology relates to hypothesis testing for the purpose of establishing cause-and-effect relationships. In the quantitative methodology, the locus of interpretation is based in mathematics or statistics. However, it is important to know that mathematical truths do not rely on experience or objects outside their own problem. Their arguments are contained within their own logic and are legitimated by the process of reasoning (Musgrave, 1993; Jarvis, 1999). Figure 2.3 illustrates the position of quantitative research, as realist ontology is the core of the positivist school of thought.

So far we have discussed one epistemological position that has maintained supremacy for almost two centuries. In the twentieth century another school of thought arose which challenged the positivist epistemology of the Enlightenment project. This is known as the interpretivist school of thought.

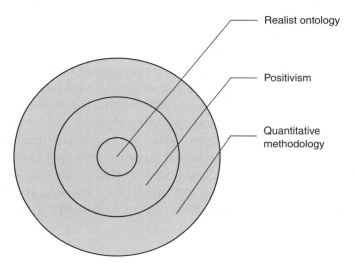

Realist ontology

Positivism

Quantitative
methodology

Figure 2.3   The relationship of realist ontology, epistemology (positivism) and quantitative methodology

2.3.2.2 The interpretivist school of thought

The main tenet in this school of thought is that the study of knowledge of humanity cannot be modelled on physical sciences; nor can we ultimately rely on and apply objective knowledge to all situations. This school of thought is seen as holistic (Crookes and Davis, 2004; Polit and Beck, 2006; Willis, 2007). In terms of research, it provides the basis for all qualitative methodology. 'Scientific knowledge cannot know and make known that it is true knowledge without resorting to other narrative kinds of knowledge' (Lyotard, 1984: 29).

Here we see another way in which we ought to understand and seek knowledge. The fundamental assertion of the interpretivist school of thought is that there is more than one reality and that these realities are constructed by the people inhabiting the world. Therefore, individuals are central to research methodology and indeed are the subject of knowledge. People are those who know about the world that they inhabit. Reality is always conditioned by our experiences, culture, beliefs and the way these are passed on to us (Guba, 1990). In keeping with the interpretivist school of thought, research ought to be conducted in the natural setting, which is not controlled by the researcher. In other words, research takes place in real-life or authentic situations (Burns and Grove, 2001; Crookes and Davies, 2004; Willis, 2007). Unlike the positivist school of thought, the interpretivist researcher is not detached but is directly involved with the people from whom and about whom knowledge is being sought (Leininger, 1985). The following example illustrates this point.

Student Example 2.2 Interpretivism

Remember James, the senior nurse in Chapter 1? He was interested in discovering the psychological impact of stoma surgery on patients and their carers. He was particularly interested in the changes in the patients' body image. James was directly involved in collecting data by talking to both stoma patients and their families. These are patients who had undergone stoma surgery and James had cared for them in the past.

This example underlines the essence of interpretivism, as the researcher (James) was able to gather a wealth of information provided by people he is researching.

From the above example you should find that there is more than one epistemological position on conducting research. The interpretivist's epistemology, from which all qualitative methodology originates, seeks to understand experience primarily from the person's perspective – the person being the subject of study. Hence the interpretivist is not concerned with facts, but with meaning and how people construe it. As you have learned in Chapter 1, qualitative research focuses on abstract concepts, such as feelings, perceptions, attitudes, values and beliefs. Thus, it is about the subjective world. Qualitative research therefore uses small-scale studies. There are two important factors that you need to consider here:

- The subjective nature of qualitative research
- The contextual nature of qualitative research.

However, as depicted in Tables 2.1 and 2.2, the scope of knowledge is wide and it is important to recognize that there are multiple sources of knowledge. The interpretivist epistemology situates the construction of knowledge in the relativist ontological orientation. Figure 2.4 illustrates the position of qualitative research, as relativist ontology is the core of the interpretivist school of thought.

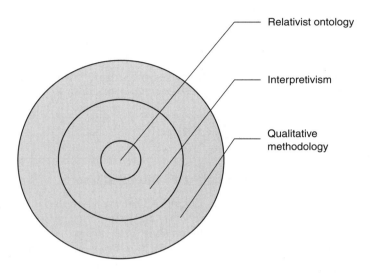

Relativist ontology

Interpretivism

Qualitative methodology

Figure 2.4   The relationship of relativist ontology, epistemology (interpretivism) and qualitative methodology

Positivism and interpretivism should not be considered as competing paradigms. They need to be looked at in connection with the intention of the research. Sometimes a particular research problem cannot be solved by resorting to either ontological and epistemological positions. In this case, a combination of each approach might be necessary. This is called mixed methodology, which was described in Chapter 1. Figure 2.5 helps to pinpoint the philosophical position of mixed methodology. This will be elaborated upon in Chapter 3 when the comprehensive review research design is described in detail.

As you have seen, the scope of knowledge is so vast that it should not be subjected to one epistemological school of thought (paradigm). When considering the research problem, it is important to have an open mind on the most appropriate choice of methodology. In the following section, we apply the issues of ontology and epistemology discussed above to the initiation of your research study.

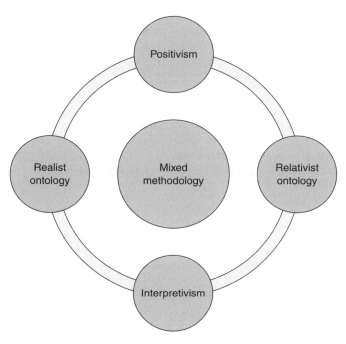

Figure 2.5 The relationship of positivism and interpretivism and mixed methodology

2.4 Shaping the purpose and scope of your research

In this section we will guide you into ways of identifying a research problem and formulating a research question. As you have learned in Chapter 1, 'research seeks answers to questions in an orderly and systematic way' (Polit and Hungler, 1999; Bluett and Cluff, 2000; Parahoo, 2006). Research must begin by clearly charting the process by which you will seek answers to the identified problem. This process needs to reflect your decision of how it ought to be conducted by considering the wider context of ontology and epistemology.

2.4.1 Identifying the research topic

This is part of the initial process of making the decision about methodological choice and design. All research begins with careful consideration of the research topic and constitutes a series of steps. It is vital to think through and ask yourself some preliminary questions about the subject and process of your research, as follows:

- What exactly are you going to research?
- Where will you obtain ideas for the proposed topic?
- How do you confirm the feasibility of your research?

The exercise below will help you unpick the subject of your research and begin the process of inquiry.

---

1 Write a sentence about your research topic.
2 Ask the following questions about your own position:

- What are my own beliefs about the topic?
- How do these influence the way I propose to conduct my study?

3 Why is the subject important?

Share your answers with another student and discuss the findings in relation to your philosophical underpinnings, as stated in the first part of this chapter.

The next step begins with looking at where you might obtain ideas for your research project. The most common place might be in the practice setting. Other sources may include something that you have read in the literature or any theories you have come across in the past (Polit and Beck, 2006). We suggest that you start with the basic step of considering what is going on around you in your practice setting. This may be to do with the evidence that is used to guide practice or, more aptly, certain aspects of nursing or midwifery care. It may be a way of doing things that you have questioned and wish to look into more deeply. You may also have had an experience that prompts you to investigate. To explore this subject of interest, you need to be aware of any presuppositions or biases and set them aside. In our experience, some students have tended to base their arguments on what they believe to be right without disputing its origins. The student example below illustrates this point.

Student Example 2.3   Identifying a research topic using personal experience

Read the following examples of students who have used their own experiences in identifying research topics.

Example (A) of a tentative research topic on the impact of mentorship on students' learning in clinical practice

Ben is a nursing student in the final year of his degree. He has had very positive learning experiences in most of his clinical learning placements. However, this

---

has not been the case with some of his fellow students as their experiences have been less conducive to learning. He cannot understand why his peers were having the problems they claimed to be having, so he became increasingly interested in researching this topic. He decided to use both his experience and that of his peers as a springboard to develop his idea. While Ben is very clear that he has his own biases, he decides not to allow this to pre-empt what his research might find.

Example (B) of a tentative research topic looking at the experience of women who have given birth at home

Jasmine is a final-year student midwife working on the delivery suite. She is dissatisfied with what she has observed about the women's birthing experience there. In a previous clinical placement she had the privilege of observing and assisting women giving birth in their natural home environment. Not only did she notice that women in their home seemed more in control, but the women themselves reported positive experiences. Adding to what she has seen in practice, Jasmine herself had her baby at home; a birth experience that was very fulfilling and, according to her story, very conducive to the successful bonding with her own baby and subsequent nurturing. In a tutorial with her research supervisor, Jasmine was convinced that her research was going to find that home is the place where women should give birth.

From the above student examples you will notice that it is important not to allow what you have observed in practice, your values and beliefs to pre-empt what your findings will be. It is good practice to start by reflecting upon the clinical and/or personal experiences that are causes for concern. This will enable you to separate the issues clearly.

STUDENT ACTIVITY 2.5

Now, to further develop your research topic, reflect on an aspect of care that you have observed in practice that interests you. The following questions will help you with your reflection:

- What is the evidence upon which the aspect of care is based?
- How was the evidence arrived at? In other words, what types of research methodology were used to arrive at this evidence?
- Look at the protocol/guidelines that tell you how to carry out the particular aspect of care. Do they represent the client's reality?
- Identify all the issues surrounding your proposed topic. What are the controversies?
- Give the reasons why you should research this chosen topic.

When you meet with your research supervisor bring these reflective notes with you. They will be very useful in structuring your initial tutorial.

To summarize, it is important for you, the researcher, to make the steps of the research process clear. The factors discussed in this section are fundamental to the rigour of your research (this will be further explored in Chapters 5 and 7). The next section discusses the relationship of professionals' and clients' ways of knowing in deciding the scope of your research project.

2.4.2 Defining the scope of your research project: seeking colleagues' and clients' perspectives

The choice of the topic for research will be largely dictated by your interest in it, but there are other pointers that should be taken into consideration. These are:

- There should be sufficient resources and literature written about the topic
- The subject should be important enough to impact on clinical decisions in practice.

Sometimes you may even think of the solution before you have conducted your research, as Student Example 2.3 (B) illustrates. For this reason it is also good practice to talk to others about your intended topic and to seek other peoples' perspectives before embarking on your research project. As we stated earlier, in any area of practice different professionals work collaboratively to provide the best care, and many of these professionals may be actively engaged in research. As each of these professionals comes from a different ontological standpoint, they may offer a fresh perspective. So you may want to talk to relevant members of the multidisciplinary team that you work with, clients and fellow students, along with your supervisor or personal tutor. At the same time, look out for conferences that are relevant to your topic as you may want to attend and talk to others, in particular those who are disseminating their own research.

▬▬▬▬ STUDENT ACTIVITY 2.6 ▬▬▬▬

- Talk to a fellow student, mentor and/or someone else from another discipline. This could be a doctor or other healthcare professional depending on the topic you are investigating.
- Make reflective notes on what you have heard, compare them with your initial observations and note down the responses which fit or contradict with your own views.
- Ask yourself what the role of talking and listening to other people's perspective is in relation to your own proposed topic of inquiry.
- Check again if there are any biases on your part.
- Compare what you have found with the philosophical discussion and the ways of knowing discussed in Student Activity 2.4.

To summarize, examining what you have found will enable you to consider the wider issues regarding your research study. Let us use an analogy from photography to illustrate the point. As Willis (2007) claims, it is like taking a picture with a wide angle lens which enables you to capture more, rather than less, of everything happening at the time. It is not only unmanageable but also imprudent to keep a wide focus as the amount of information may be inappropriate and/or superficial. You should now 'zoom in' to focus on the specific area you wish to explore. An exploration of the literature will contribute towards achieving a manageable focus.

2.4.3 Defining the scope of your research project: exploring the literature

As in empirical research, initial exploration of the literature (in the literature review methodology) is an essential part of the research process as the work of others will inform and establish your own (Hart, 1998). Exploring the literature will allow you to find out what is already known about the subject and the areas of deficiencies. In so doing, you will build on the picture that has already started to emerge during the previous exercise (Student Activity 2.6). You will also seek to find new perspectives from the literature and discover what makes your study unique and authentic.

What you choose to include in your initial exploration of literature will be dependent on your area of study. However, you may organize your literature review in terms of empirical and non-empirical sources of literature (see Figure 2.6).

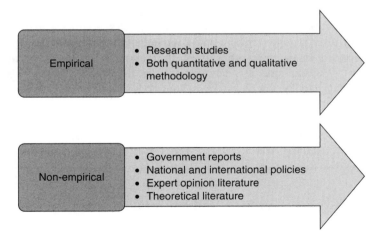

Figure 2.6 Types of empirical and non-empirical sources of literature

A question that our students have frequently asked us is how many studies they need to search and review? There is no clear-cut answer to this question; however, there are questions you may ask that will help you define how far you go with your literature review:

- What evidence do I need to establish if my topic is worth researching?
- Is there any research that has been done on my topic? (If there is scant literature, it may be difficult to complete your research project.)

The following student example illustrates this point.

Student Example 2.4   Exploring the literature

After talking to the specialist nurse in diabetes on Donna's last clinical placement area, she has decided that diabetes adherence is the topic of interest for her final-year research project. Donna explores the literature by conducting an initial literature review using the keywords 'diabetes' and 'adherence to treatment and advice' in the *Google Scholar* search engine. She discovers the following journal article:

Hearnshaw, H. and Lindenmeyer, A. (2006) 'What do we mean by adherence to treatment and advice for living with diabetes? A review of the literature on definitions and measurements', *Diabetic Medicine*, 23(7), 720–728.

This journal was invaluable as the authors reviewed 293 published papers on the topic. Donna was able to obtain and read some of the publications. She found that some of the research findings coincided with her personal experience of nursing diabetic patients in the past. However, several of these articles are quite old so she needs to search for more current literature on the subject.

The above example demonstrates the importance of keeping an open mind on the topic of interest when conducting your initial literature review. The use of concise keywords helps, as do other search strategies that will be elaborated upon in Chapter 4. This example also demonstrates another important point, which is the use of published literature reviews on your chosen topic. However, although it may seem an efficient way of reviewing the literature on your topic, it can also be misleading because literature review articles may not necessarily cover the exact area you are exploring. Always refer back to your mind-map(s) and research aims and objectives, as these help to remind you of your defined parameters.

To summarize, what you need to constantly bear in mind is the remit of your research and that one of the purposes of the literature review is to narrow your focus. The next section addresses this difficult task.

2.4.4 Narrowing your topic

Bear in mind that while the subject in its entirety may be so interesting that scoping (or defining the parameters of your research) it may be an indefinite task, your research project needs to be completed. So it is worth remembering that too broad a topic will consume a lot of your time and energy. This will prevent you from achieving the level of depth that the research requires. In my own quest for understanding what midwifery is, which has been an area of great interest to me for a number of years, my initial research title was 'Midwifery and Globalization'. This was clearly unmanageable for a relatively new researcher. After reflecting on the topic, talking to others, reading around the vast subject, developing my own conceptual framework and creating a mind-map, I decided that my real interest was in seeking to understand the development of midwifery knowledge – a focus that was much more manageable.

In the process of making up your mind and talking to others, you may eventually have some pointers with regards to the specific area that you want to look at. The most important rules that you need to keep in mind and that will dictate the scope of your research project are:

- The time frame: ask yourself how long you have to complete your project
- The word limit: find out how much you need to write
- The area or topic of research: this needs to be manageable and determined by the context of practice in which you want to make a contribution.

2.5 Formulating and refining your research question or statement

You may have started to search into your topic by asking yourself a question or writing down a statement. Many students start that way. It is necessary to ensure that your question is answerable and the statement is precise. It may therefore take a few attempts to get it just right. Formulating an answerable question or a concise statement entails engaging with and critically reading the literature (Clough and Nutbrown, 2000; O'Brien and Pipkin, 2007). We cannot emphasize enough how important it is to have the right question or statement, for it is your research question or statement that will be the 'navigator in the ship' of your research or, if you prefer, the 'pilot in the aeroplane' of your research. A frequent and valid question that our students have asked is 'How do I write a research question or statement?' There are two ways of doing so. It can be either a declarative statement or an interrogative question (Aveyard, 2010):

1 A *declarative* statement may help you stay focused as you are stating the intention of your research. It will give you a clear direction for your study. This is particularly useful if you are taking a deductive approach. An example of this is: *An exploration of the influence of media on women's perception of home birth*. However, the disadvantage is that you are less likely to look beyond what is stated.
2 An *interrogative* question, on the other hand, may lead you away from the research focus, luring you into other directions or perspectives of the topic under exploration. An example of this is: *What is the relationship between perceptions of home birth in the media and women's perception of home birth?* However, the strength of using a research question is that you have kept an open and unbiased mind. This is particularly useful if you are coming from an inductive approach to research.

STUDENT ACTIVITY 2.7

This activity draws together what you have learned from yourself and others so as to formulate a declarative statement or an interrogative research question.

Writing a research statement

If you have decided on a deductive approach to your research – that is, the intention of your research is clear – a research statement will be more apt. A research statement is a complete sentence that states clearly your topic of interest, the target population and, if possible, where the research is conducted (e.g. a hospital, community setting or university). Research statements can sometimes be written as a set of objectives.

Now try and write one or several research statement(s) to suit your topic.

Formulating a research question

If you have decided on an inductive approach to your research – that is, the outcome of the research is uncertain – a research question will be more suitable. Research questions, if written correctly, need be open questions. In other words, if your research question can be answered by a simple 'yes' or 'no', then it is likely that you have pre-empted the outcome of your research and perhaps a research statement is more suitable. Yin (2003) states that research questions should be 'what', 'how' or 'why' questions.

Now, try and write a research question to suit your topic.

Bring these with you when you meet with your research supervisor. They will be very useful in structuring your tutorials.

Now that you have formulated your research question/statement, you are in a position to situate your research within a wider philosophical and methodological framework. The flowchart in Figure 2.7, which is adapted from Clough and Nutbrown (2000), brings together the stages involved in your research.

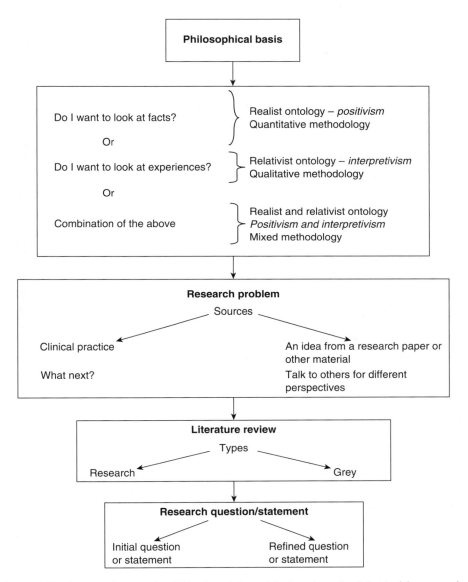

Figure 2.7 Stages of research within the philosophical and methodological framework

End-of-Chapter Learning Points

We hope that you have found this chapter helpful in understanding the wider philosophical underpinning of research and how the choice of appropriate methodology is made. The following are the key points highlighted in this chapter:

1 There are different types of knowledge that may be important in nursing and midwifery, especially now that most healthcare settings serve a population from diverse backgrounds. In addition, nursing and midwifery knowledge bases are informed by other disciplines.
2 Research is not just about methodology and methods. It has to be anchored on a wider philosophical underpinning. Indeed, there are different philosophical bases that may undergird a research design. This is dependent upon the school of thought within which the researchers are socialized and to which they subscribe. Most important of all, the different schools of thought – that is, positivism and interpretivism – should not be viewed as contending paradigms. Each serves its purpose for the knowledge being sought.
3 Identifying a research problem, although complex, is an exciting part of the research process that enables the chosen research topic to be explored from different peoples' perspectives. A critical interpretation of the topic is therefore required.
4 Literature review is also an important part of the research process because it enables you to narrow the focus of the study. It should indicate what has already been researched, how it has been researched and where there are gaps in your proposed subject.
5 Any research project needs a research question or a statement. This is what guides the research. It needs to be focused.

References

On philosophy

Chalmers, A. (1990) *Science and its Fabrication*. Minneapolis, MN: University of Minnesota Press.
Descartes, R. (1968) *Discourse on Method and Mediations*. Translated by F.E. Sutcliffe. London: Penguin (originally published 1637).
Jarvis, P. (1999) *The Practitioner-Researcher: Developing Theory from Practice*. San Francisco, CA: Jossey-Bass.

Lyotard, J. (1984) *The Postmodern Condition: A Report on Knowledge*. Manchester: Manchester University Press.

Musgrave, A. (1993) *Common Sense, Science and Scepticism: A Historical Introduction to the Theory of Knowledge*. Cambridge: Cambridge University Press.

On research

Aveyard, H. (2010) *Doing a Literature Review in Health and Social Care* (2nd edn). Maidenhead: Open University Press.

Bluett, E.R. and Cluff, R. (2000) *Principles and Practice of Research in Midwifery*. Edinburgh: Bailliere Tindall.

Burns, N. and Grove, S.K. (2001) *The Practice of Nursing Research* (4th edn). Philadelphia, PA: W.B. Saunders.

Clough, P. and Nutbrown, C. (2000) *A Student's Guide to Methodology*. London: Sage.

Crookes, A. and Davies, S. (eds) (2004) *Research into Practice* (2nd edn). Edinburgh: Bailliere Tindall.

Denzin, N.K. and Lincoln, Y.S. (eds) (1998) *Strategies of Qualitative Inquiry*. Thousand Oaks, CA: Sage.

Guba, E.G. (1990) *The Paradigm Dialogue*. London: Sage.

Hart, C. (1998) *Doing a Literature Review: Releasing the Social Science Research Imagination*. London: Sage.

Leininger, M.M. (ed.) (1985) *Qualitative Research Methods in Nursing*. Orlando, FL: Grune and Stratton.

O'Brien, P.M.S. and Pipkin, F.B. (2007) *Introduction to Research Principles for Specialist and Trainees* (2nd edn). London: RCOG Press.

Parahoo, K. (2006) *Nursing Research: Principles, Process and Issues* (2nd edn). Basingstoke: Palgrave Macmillan.

Paterson, B.L., Thorne, S.E., Canam, C. and Jillings, C. (2001) *Meta-Study of Qualitative Health Research*. Thousand Oaks, CA: Sage.

Polit, D.F. and Hungler, B.P. (1999) *Nursing Research: Principles and Methods*. Philadelphia: Lippincott Williams/Wilkins.

Polit, D.F. and Beck, C.T. (2006) *Essentials of Nursing Research: Methods, Appraisal and Utilization* (6th edn). Philadelphia, PA: Lippincott, Williams & Wilkins.

Willis, J.W. (2007) *Foundations of Qualitative Research*. Thousand Oaks, CA: Sage.

Yin, R.K. (2003) *Case Study Research: Design and Methods* (3rd edn). London: Sage.

On diabetes

Hearnshaw, H. and Lindenmeyer, A. (2006) 'What do we mean by adherence to treatment and advice for living with diabetes? A review of the literature on definitions and measurements', *Diabetic Medicine*, 23(7), 720–728.

THREE

Research Design: Comprehensive Literature Review as a Research Methodology

---

Aim and objectives

The aim of this chapter is to introduce the principles underpinning literature review methodology design. By the end of this chapter you will be able to:

- Differentiate between empirical and non-empirical research designs
- Understand literature review as a research methodology and be familiar with the process involved in designing a comprehensive literature review
- Justify literature review as a methodology in its own right
- Design a comprehensive literature review research project.

3.1 Introduction

In the previous chapter, we explored the philosophical basis of research from an empirical standpoint. We now focus on literature-based research methodology and its relationship to its ontological and epistemological underpinning. Literature review methodology has long been recognized as an important methodological approach to solve research problems. Streubert and Carpenter (2011) consider this non-empirical methodology to be critical for advancing and developing new insight into nursing and midwifery knowledge. In most academic research texts, literature review is defined as part of the process involved in empirical research. Explicitly, a literature review is used to uncover what is already known about a subject before the actual study begins (Hart, 1998). To a large extent this is true, but literature review as methodology goes beyond this process. So, it is important to differentiate between literature review as part of the process of empirical research and as a research methodology in its own right. In this chapter we show that designing a comprehensive literature review (as a type of literature review methodology) involves the same process as designing empirical research. The philosophical root of both empirical and non-empirical research is compared in Figure 3.1.

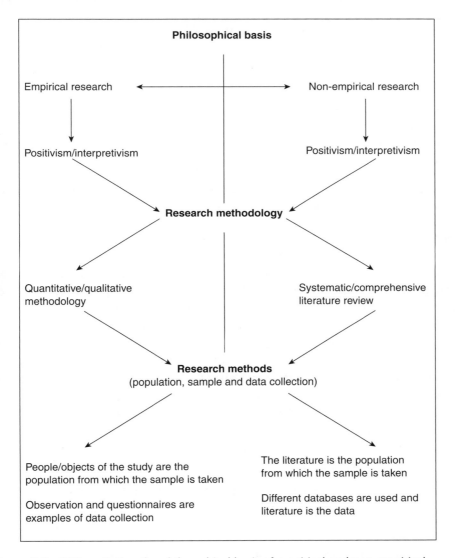

Figure 3.1 Differentiating the philosophical basis of empirical and non-empirical research

The key issue in non-empirical research is that the researcher works with data that someone else has collected for a particular purpose and presented in research reports. For your study, you will be following the non-empirical route illustrated in Figure 3.1.

3.2 Literature review: a research methodology

Terms such as 'systematic review', 'integrated review' (Whittemore and Knafl, 2005; Cooper, 2010; Jesson et al., 2011), 'narrative review' (Green et al. 2006) and 'qualitative review' (Centre for Reviews and Dissemination, 2009) are used to describe literature review methodology. The key distinguishing features in the literature review methodology compared with empirical research design are:

- The literature is the population that provides the data for the study
- The sample comes from the literature
- Data collection in the research setting is conducted by searching through the various databases
- The analysis is based on clear evaluative criteria
- The findings are synthesized using a systematic approach (such as meta-analysis, meta-synthesis, meta-ethnography and meta-theory).

Traditionally, the emphasis of literature review research design has been on the systematic review of either quantitative or qualitative research literature. Reviews of quantitative research literature are seen as rigorous (Higgins and Green, 2011; Jesson et al., 2011). In contrast, qualitative literature reviews are frequently criticized for lacking the clear-cut steps in their design; that is 'the studies found are identified by chance rather than in a systematic way' (Centre for Reviews and Dissemination, 2009: 252) and for not yielding reliable evidence (Petticrew and Roberts, 2006). The pluralist approach of reviewing both quantitative and qualitative research plus grey literature has received little attention. Popay (2006) has attempted to address this imbalance, although her publication, under the auspice of the National Institute for Health and Clinical Excellence (NICE) is more appropriate for fully-fledged, experienced researchers. Our aim in this book is to guide you through a rigorous process of designing a comprehensive literature review for your research project.

3.3 Types of literature review methodology

Literature review methodology can be categorized under two main headings:

- Systematic review of mainly quantitative research of similar designs
- Comprehensive literature review of quantitative/qualitative research papers, mixed methodology research design and grey literature.

Your choice of methodology, as discussed in Chapter 2, will depend on what answers your research question/statement seeks to explore. Some research questions or statements cannot be answered within the two discrete philosophical positions of positivism and interpretivism (as illustrated in Figure 3.1). Often there may be a need to combine or mix both methodologies. Several authors have acknowledged the contribution of mixed methodologies to understanding evidence (Denzin and Lincoln, 1998; Brannen, 2005; Sheldon, 2005; Polit and Beck, 2006).

The common ground in both systematic and comprehensive literature review methodologies is simply this: they both utilize existing literature for the following stages of the research process:

- Sampling
- Data collection
- Data analysis and synthesis

Although this chapter is not about how to undertake a systematic review, a brief overview is given to enable you to familiarize yourself with the process involved in conducting research in which mainly quantitative literature is used as data.

3.3.1 Systematic review

A systematic review is a quantitative research methodology. In effect, it is a research of research by reviewing mainly quantitative research papers of similar designs. Some definitions of the term 'systematic review' are given below:

> A scientific tool which can be used to summarize, appraise and communicate the results and implications of otherwise unmanageable quantities of research. (NHS Centre for Reviews and Dissemination, 2009: v, www.york.ac.uk/inst/crd/pdf/Systematic_Review.pdf)

> The rigorous search, selection, appraisal, synthesis and summary of the findings of primary research in order to answer a specific question. (Parahoo, 2006: 134)

> A review in which all the evidence pertaining to a particular field of research has been collected via a systematic search of the literature and unpublished sources and evaluated using predefined quality criteria. (O'Brien and Pipkin, 2007: 59)

Systematic reviews attempt to collate all empirical evidence and use prespecified eligibility criteria in order to answer a specific research statement (hypothesis) or question. They use explicit, systematic methods that are selected with a view to minimizing bias, thus providing more reliable findings from which conclusions can be drawn and decisions made (Antman et al., 1992; Oxman, 1994).

Liberati et al. (2009: W65) state that systematic reviews and meta-analyses are essential tools for summarizing evidence accurately and reliably. There are at least 2,500 new systematic reviews reported in English and they are indexed in *Medline* annually. Liberati et al. highlight the strengths of systematic reviews as follows:

- They provide clinicians with a quick reference for clinical decisions
- They use explicit methods which limits bias in providing conclusions that are more reliable and accurate
- They provide evidence for healthcare providers, researchers and policy makers to appraise risks, benefits and harms of interventions
- They collate and summarize related research for patients and healthcare practitioners/carers
- They assist clinical practitioners in developing evidence-based guidelines.

STUDENT ACTIVITY 3.1

Go into *The Cochrane Handbook* (2011), which is available at www.cochrane-handbook. org, and identify the characteristics of a systematic review. Share your findings with another student and keep these notes at hand for the next exercise.

3.3.1.1 The steps involved in conducting a systematic review

Conducting a systematic review requires a definite structure based on a prespecified number of stepwise criteria. These are as follows:

Set a clear research question
↓
Search the evidence and define the inclusion criteria
↓
Assess the validity of the papers by critical appraisal and assessment of risk
↓
Extract and assess the quality of the data and synthesize the data
↓
Disseminate the findings

3.3.1.2 Method of data analysis in a systematic review

The most common method of analysis for systematic reviews is called meta-analysis. Often the term meta-analysis is used synonymously with systematic reviews. Meta-analysis is a statistical technique for analyzing quantitative studies and is mainly a set of procedures that are used to statistically combine the findings of a number of quantitative research studies. Sackett et al. (1997) state that meta-analysis consists of systematic review incorporating a specific statistical strategy for assembling the results of several studies into a single estimate.

Some of the advantages of a meta-analysis are as follows:

- It increases the power of the statistical findings because of greater numbers
- It improves precision as findings are based on the combination of results of several studies. This gives a more reliable and precise estimate of the effectiveness of interventions than a stand-alone study
- It answers questions that have not been posed by the original studies
- It settles controversies that have arisen from apparent conflicting studies or generates new hypotheses. (Higgins and Green, 2011)

Meta-analysis is important because a large number of research studies, even though they have employed a rigorous design, may lack statistical power to show significant effect. Systematic reviews are able to help decision makers cope with the volume of studies by summarizing them as well as providing 'new' information which may not be apparent from individual studies, particularly where the effects under investigation are small. If a study is using a small number of participants or there is a small difference between the intervention and the control groups, it is difficult to assign much significance to the result. However, if similar studies are combined, the results become much more powerful as they are based on larger numbers. A lot of trust, therefore, is placed in systematic reviews and clinicians rely on them more and more when making decisions about treatment and the management of patients and clients.

STUDENT ACTIVITY 3.2

Read the following abstract which is taken from a published systematic review undertaken by Ndosi et al. (2011) and address the questions below.

Objectives

The objective of this systematic review was to determine the effectiveness of nurse-led care in rheumatoid arthritis.

Design

Systematic review of effectiveness.

Data sources

Electronic databases (AMED, CENTRAL, CINAHL, EMBASE, HMIC, HTA, MEDLINE, NHEED, Ovid Nursing and PsycINFO) were searched from 1988 to January 2010

(Continued)

with no language restrictions. Inclusion criteria were: randomized controlled trials, nurse-led care being part of the intervention and including patients with RA.

Review methods

Data were extracted by one reviewer and checked by a second reviewer. Quality assessment was conducted independently by two reviewers using the Cochrane Collaboration's Risk of Bias Tool. For each outcome measure, the effect size was assessed using risk ratio or ratio of means (RoM) with corresponding 95% confidence intervals (CI) as appropriate. Where possible, data from similar outcomes were pooled in a meta-analysis.

Results

Seven records representing four randomized controlled trials (RCTs) with an overall low risk of bias (good quality) were included in the review. They included 431 patients and the interventions (nurse-led care vs usual care) lasted for 1–2 years. Most effect sizes of disease activity measures were inconclusive (DAS28 RoM = 0.96, 95%CI [0.90–1.02], $P = 0.16$; plasma viscosity RoM = 1, 95%CI [0.8–1.26], $P = 0.99$) except the Ritchie Articular Index (RoM = 0.89, 95%CI [0.84–0.95], $P < 0.001$) which favoured nurse-led care. Results from some secondary outcomes (functional status, stiffness and coping with arthritis) were also inconclusive. Other outcomes (satisfaction and pain) displayed mixed results when assessed using different tools making them also inconclusive. Significant effects of nurse-led care were seen in quality of life (RAQoL RoM = 0.83, 95%CI [0.75–0.92], $P < 0.001$), patient knowledge (PKQ RoM = 4.39, 95%CI [3.35–5.72], $P < 0.001$) and fatigue (median difference = −330, $P = 0.02$).

Conclusions

The estimates of the primary outcome and most secondary outcomes showed no significant difference between nurse-led care and the usual care. While few outcomes favoured nurse-led care, there is insufficient evidence to conclude whether this is the case. More good quality RCTs of nurse-led care effectiveness in rheumatoid arthritis are required.

Discuss with another student the characteristics of a systematic review as defined by *The Cochrane Handbook* (2011) and answer the following questions:

- Were the search criteria clearly stated?
- What numbers in the sample (literature reviewed) were included in the meta-analysis?
- Did the result and conclusion reflect the initial objectives set for the review?

We hope you find in your discussion that the process of conducting a systematic review is arduous and thorough! The researcher needs to have a sound knowledge of statistics or else a statistician must be at hand to give advice.

3.3.2 The comprehensive literature review:
an overview of the process and four key principles

Comprehensive review is a literature review methodology which aims to provide you with a pluralistic approach to conducting your research. The strength of the comprehensive literature review is that it uses an array of literature (published quantitative, qualitative and mixed methodology research as well as grey literature). The use of a combination of positivist and interpretivist paradigms provides added rigour, hence the term 'comprehensive'. This literature review methodology provides the depth that is required as the combination of empirical and non-empirical literature selected for review complements each other. In what follows, we will show you how to design a comprehensive literature review that parallels empirical research both in design and methodological rigour. This is illustrated in Figure 3.2.

Following the model in Figure 3.2 will allow you to demonstrate a structured and iterative approach to designing your comprehensive literature review. Simply following this approach can clarify the research topic itself, from defining your research problem and formulating a precise research question/statement through to undertaking a clear and unbiased synthesis of your research findings and culminating in a research report. This process approach to the design of the comprehensive literature review demonstrates that it is a methodology in its own right (Crotty, 2003). The iterative processes allow you to go back and forth when considering the stages of your research. It takes you through the intricate steps of examining your philosophical position when deciding on the use of the mixed methodological approach. This in turn will help you to construct meaningful research question(s) and statement(s) that will guide you through the rest of the research stages. Similarly, while in the course of collecting and critiquing the literature, you may wish to back-track and re-examine your methodology and research question/statement. Even when you are embarking on the analysis and synthesis of themes, there may be a need to collect more literature that will open up avenues not previously considered.

There are four key principles that underpin the theoretical framework of the comprehensive literature review methodology. These are:

1 The researcher's ontological and epistemological stance need to be explicit (see section 3.4).
2 Data are generated through a pluralistic approach (see section 3.5).
3 There is a formal process of critique for data analysis (see section 3.6).
4 The researcher must be ethically aware of the need for rigour throughout the whole research process (see section 3.7).

The rest of this chapter will be devoted to defining the comprehensive literature review research design in accordance with the above principles.

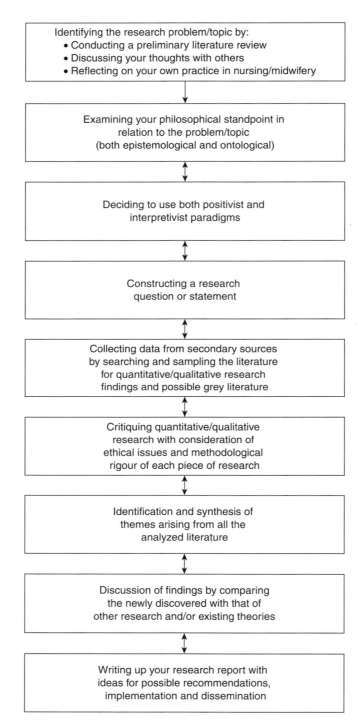

Identifying the research problem/topic by:
• Conducting a preliminary literature review
• Discussing your thoughts with others
• Reflecting on your own practice in nursing/midwifery

Examining your philosophical standpoint in
relation to the problem/topic
(both epistemological and ontological)

Deciding to use both positivist and
interpretivist paradigms

Constructing a research
question or statement

Collecting data from secondary sources
by searching and sampling the literature
for quantitative/qualitative research
findings and possible grey literature

Critiquing quantitative/qualitative
research with consideration of
ethical issues and methodological
rigour of each piece of research

Identification and synthesis of
themes arising from all the
analyzed literature

Discussion of findings by comparing
the newly discovered with that of
other research and/or existing theories

Writing up your research report with
ideas for possible recommendations,
implementation and dissemination

Figure 3.2   A model defining the research process in the design of the comprehensive
literature review

DOING A RESEARCH PROJECT IN NURSING & MIDWIFERY

3.4 Principle 1: The researcher's ontological and epistemological stance needs to be explicit

All research needs to be situated within a solid philosophical framework to determine what data the researcher should seek. Your comprehensive literature review is no different. The philosophical underpinning is the backbone of any research study and should guide the research design from beginning to end. You have already learned that it is the first step in designing your research project. As discussed in Chapter 2, there are two main ontological and epistemological stances:

- Positivism
- Interpretivism

These philosophical underpinnings represent different ways of looking at knowledge and thereby informing research methodology. Merriam (2001) claims that philosophical underpinnings are an important aspect of research design. Researchers bring to a research project their own philosophical perspectives that shape the research design. These philosophical underpinnings come from the same three contexts discussed in Chapter 2 (see Figure 3.3).

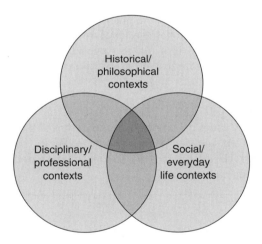

Figure 3.3   The contexts of belief systems (adapted from Paterson et al., 2001)

   The significance of philosophical underpinnings is that they should link the research question/statement to much wider issues, such as policy issues (Marshall and Rossman, 1995). Therefore it is important that these are made explicit.

   In a comprehensive literature review, the researcher recognizes that the design may encompass broader philosophical underpinnings. It enables the inclusion of data that do not fit in just one philosophical position. Your research statement/question may necessitate that you investigate your topic from different vantage points. Thus, in designing a comprehensive literature review, you, the researcher, will base the design on a combination of interpretivism and positivism; hence, it is a pluralistic approach. If your research seeks to understand human experiences, then an interpretivist stance will suffice. But if, in addition to human experiences, you want to know about the impact of intervention tools, then it will be appropriate to combine both stances. You may also need to think about your own biases; it would be good practice to declare these at the outset of your research.

Student Example 3.1   Philosophical underpinnings of the researcher

Jane is a researcher from a pharmaceutical company working on the subject of 'Patients'/clients' attitudes to pain'. Jane's initial exploration of the literature on the subject of pain leads her to an array of qualitative research on clients' pain experiences.

However, she is also interested in the use of pain relief and how it affects clients' attitudes to pain. Further literature search has resulted in clinical trials of clients' attitudes to traditional and complementary pain relief methods. These quantitative research studies utilized attitudinal scales and pain scores to measure client outcomes.

The funding of her research from the pharmaceutical company has enabled her to submit a proposal for a comprehensive literature review to encompass both qualitative and quantitative data over a ten-year period. She is particularly interested in comparing research undertaken with client groups, such as those undergoing surgery and childbirth.

From this example you will notice that:

- Funding and policy issues govern the size and design of the project
- Jane's experience and knowledge allows her to widen the scope of her search
- The topic 'Patients'/clients' attitudes to pain' needs to be pared down to a workable research statement/question.

3.5 Principle 2: Data is generated through a pluralistic approach

This section focuses on the type of data that is required to answer your research question/statement in order to reflect the pluralistic nature of your design. It is important to remember that the literature is the data and it can be vast. So your next step is to specify your target population and from there choose your sample. For a comprehensive literature review, your target population may include empirical quantitative and qualitative research papers and grey literature. When

Table 3.1 The sample frame

Quantitative research	Qualitative research	Mixed methodology research	Grey literature
Randomized controlled trials	Ethnographic studies	Mixture of research of contrasting paradigms	Audits
Quasi-experiments	Phenomenological studies	Mixture of research of the same paradigm	Government reports
Cohort studies	Grounded theory studies		Expert opinions
Surveys	Feminist or participatory studies		Theoretical literature

deciding upon the types of literature that will constitute your samples you need to make a list of what constitutes your target population (Parahoo, 2006). So a sample frame is a necessary tool in the process of sampling. The rest of this section will be devoted to exploring the sample frame, sampling methods, inclusion and exclusion criteria and data collection as a process.

3.5.1 Sample frame

The sample frame provides you with a complete coverage of the literature. A sample may be drawn from studies using similar methodology or from studies using a diversity of methodology (Cooper, 2010). Table 3.1 gives an exemplar of a sample frame.

Table 3.1 provides a picture of where you might begin to look for your sample. Choosing your sample frame is not as straightforward as it might first appear. Some empirical research may employ a combination of methods of data collection or even different philosophical approaches. These are some important considerations not only for your subject of inquiry but also when designing your sample frame. For instance, a design using mixed methodology may include both structured questionnaires and follow-up unstructured interviews. On the other hand, a pure (but mixed) qualitative design may use a combination of feminist and participatory approaches. So employing mixed methodology encompasses more than just quantitative and qualitative empirical approaches. It may also be a combination of several qualitative methodologies.

As discussed in Chapter 1, there are two types of mixed methodology research designs: the sequential or concurrent designs. In a sequential design one methodological approach informs the other, whereas in a concurrent design the quantitative and qualitative data are collected simultaneously in the same study (Denzin and Lincoln, 1998).

In summary, you may need to decide what sort of evidence will be appropriate to answer your research question and how you will manage data generation. Sampling, which we discuss in the next section, addresses these issues.

3.5.2 Sampling methods

In choosing the sampling method, you should ensure that this is achieved in a systematic, explicit and reproducible manner (Booth, 2001). Thus, if someone else follows your strategy, they will find the same set of papers (Randolph, 2009). Sample selection starts by identifying the whole population and then narrowing to the selected sample from which you will obtain data. In defining the sample it is important to grasp that this is not just a linear step in the research process but also an iterative process. Figure 3.4 provides an example of how to determine the sample.

Selecting a sample of relevant literature of the types outlined in Figure 3.4 constitutes your data. As well as making your research manageable, you will also be able to decide which types of data your research falls into in order to obtain answers/evidence that will prove useful for generating knowledge or new insight into your research problem. In his taxonomy of literature reviews,

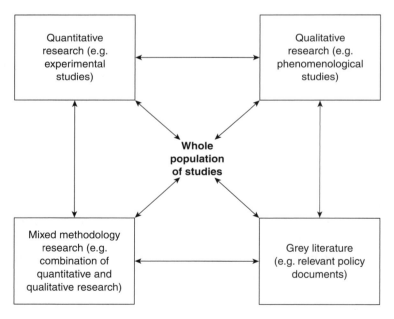

Figure 3.4   Determining the sample

Cooper (2010: 5) calls this process 'coverage' and he identifies four different types of sample:

1 **Exhaustive sample** – this includes all the literature on the research topic. (A word of caution about choosing this sample type: do consider the resources, time and scope of your study!)
2 **Exhaustive review with selective citation sample** – the researcher selects what to include from the whole population of studies.
3 **Representative sample** – a selection from the whole population that is representative of it.
4 **Central or pivotal sample** – this is the same as a purposive sample 'where participants are deliberately chosen on the basis that they can provide the necessary data' (Parahoo, 2006: 268).

▨▨▨▨▨▨▨▨▨▨▨ **STUDENT ACTIVITY 3.3** ▨▨▨▨▨▨▨▨▨▨▨

Return to your research question/statement, as written in Chapter 2, and ask yourself the following questions:

•   Which type of research studies apply to my research?
•   Which types of methodology have these research studies employed?
•   Which type of grey literature might apply to my research (see Figure 3.4 for examples of grey literature)?

Now make a list of the studies that are relevant to your research and cross-check it with your research question/statement.

Word of caution: You need to know where to stop!

From the above exercise you would have realized that sample selection is an important part of the research design. Clearly, the selection of the sample is based on your judgement, but there are at least two further considerations that are important:

• Your sample is a representative quota from your target population (very often it is at this stage that we have seen students deviating from their target population).
• The scope of your study will define which type of sample to use. This might be either of the four sampling types mentioned above.

From the list that you have compiled in Student Activity 3.3, you may find that the literature is vast. Therefore some inclusion and exclusion criteria are required in order to keep within the scope of your study. The next section explores just that.

3.5.3 Inclusion and exclusion criteria

Using inclusion and exclusion criteria, sometimes referred to as eligibility criteria, is a strategy to help specify the types of data that will best answer your research question/statement (Polit and Beck, 2006). To some extent the above section on sampling has already talked about inclusion and exclusion criteria but here we want to be more specific.

A common challenge that students face is to decide what literature ought to be included in their research project. Many students have been overwhelmed by the vast amount of literature pertaining to their topic. It is also tempting when you are collecting data to get sidetracked by captivating titles and digress from the focus of your research.(So imposing inclusion and exclusion criteria will enable you to identify literature that is relevant to your study.)

When you are deciding what to include and exclude in your study it is crucial that you have your research question/statement at hand. It is important that these criteria are carefully thought through on two counts. First, you need to avoid introducing bias into your review. Secondly, it is important to ensure that the quality of research studies and/or grey literature is enough to solve the research problem and advance knowledge (Whittemore and Knafl, 2005). Thus you need to justify your choice of inclusion and exclusion criteria, and this should be clearly documented. Table 3.2 gives an example of what a set of inclusion and exclusion criteria may look like:

Table 3.2 Exemplar of inclusion and exclusion criteria

Inclusion criteria	Exclusion criteria
Professional literature	Non-professional literature
Qualitative research with stated methodologies	Theses or dissertations
High-quality randomized controlled trials	Systematic reviews
Written in English language	Studies not written in English
Time frame – literature published between 2002 and 2010	Time frame – literature published before 2002

3.5.4 Data collection

As a continuum of research design, the method of data collection is important as it will influence the findings of your research. Thus data collection includes a series of steps and involves a well-defined strategy. We cannot emphasize enough how important a well-defined strategy for data collection is to the rigour of your research project. This process will be detailed in Chapter 4. However, the following student example introduces you to the vital step of keeping a running log of your searches as part of the data collection process.

Student Example 3.2   Log of literature searches when collecting data

Inclusion criteria

Empirical and non-empirical literature
Non-professional literature
Publications in the period 2002–2012
English language

Key

E = empirical   NE = non-empirical or grey literature
NP = non-professional literature
Search engines = G: Google, GS: Google Scholar, BNI, CINAHL
Country of origin = UK, USA, AUS, ESP, Nordic, other English-speaking
countries, etc.

Keywords

'diabetes' and 'lifestyle changes'	127 hits (NP, Google, all UK)
'nurse' and 'type II diabetes'	57 hits (E, GS, BNI, 26 USA, 13 UK, 7 AUS, 6 ESP, 5 Nordic)
'type II diabetes' and 'self management'	42 hits (E, NE, GS, BNI, 20 USA, 11 UK, 7 AUS, 4 Other)
'type II diabetes' and 'education'	38 hits (E, NE, GS, BNI, 19 UK, 18 USA)
'type II diabetes' and 'adherence'	15 hits (E, GS, CINAHL, 6 USA, 4 UK, 3 AUS, 2 Nordic)

The above log demonstrates how you can keep a summary of important information that you might refer back to later on in your research process. The key devised in this example is an exemplar which can be modified to suit the purpose of your research. In this example, non-professional literature is accessed for background reading, which can be useful as part of the initial literature review to help narrow the focus of your topic.

3.6 Principle 3: There is a formal process of critique in data analysis

Data analysis is one of the most challenging tasks in the comprehensive literature review methodology. In Chapter 5 this process will be discussed fully. This section only gives an introduction to this formal process. Although a number of research texts explore analysis of literature-based data, few provide a detailed strategy of how this is negotiated. The main consideration in the analysis of literature-based data, as Cooper (2010) points out, is judging if the data are 'trustworthy'. Therefore, it is imperative that the method of analysis is systematic and based on explicit criteria. This needs to include everything from underlying ontological and epistemological assumptions right through to data collection, all of which have implications for analysis.

There are a number of critique frameworks that you may choose to analyze data, but there may be a problem in deciding which one is the most appropriate, particularly if you are using a mixed methodology approach. A more effective way is to devise a data extraction tool (NHS Centre for Reviews and Dissemination, 2009) which allows you to create all the criteria for judging the rigour of the data you are analyzing and, at the same time, helps you determine the rigour of your own method of analysis. This is a formal process as the decision of what information to extract from the data will be dependent on your research question/statement. Table 3.3 gives an example of a well-delineated procedure of a data extraction tool.

The data extraction tool exemplified in Table 3.3 borrows from the principle of systematic review. However, in a comprehensive literature review the information that you will extract will differ from that in a systematic review – it will be dependent on the type of literature from which data are extracted. We emphasize that the data extraction tool is only a step in the analytic process. The successful extraction requires structured reading of the text on a number of occasions and is similar to reading transcribed interviews from an empirical research project. Carney's 'Ladder of Analytical Abstraction' (1990), cited in Miles and Huberman (1994: 92), is a good example to use for structured reading. It is important to have a set of questions to guide your reading as part of the data analysis and extraction process (these set questions and ideas for structured reading will be further elaborated in Chapter 5).

3.7 Principle 4: The researcher must be ethically aware of the need for rigour throughout the whole research process

Ethics is an important component of research. It is outside the scope of this section to enter into a detailed discussion of the principles of ethics and their applicability to the research process, although this has been elaborated in most academic texts on research and government policy documents. For instance, the Department of Health's *Research Governance Framework for Health and Social Care* (2001) identifies clearly the codes of ethics pertaining to research. Generally speaking, ethics can be defined as follows:

Table 3.3 Exemplar of a data extraction tool

Date	Author/ researcher	Philosophical basis	Research question	Methodology	Sample	Data collection	Data analysis	Findings	Conclusions
Paper 1									
Paper 2									
Paper 3									
Paper 4									
Paper 5									
Paper 6									
Paper 7									
Paper 8									
Paper 9									
Paper 10 etc.									

> [Ethics are] Concerned with analysing moral values and seeking to understand what people consider to be good, right, and just. It is also about what individuals consider or feel that they ought to do and about the actual way in which they behave so it is both cognitive and action-orientated. (Jarvis, 1997: 15)

> The field of ethics, also called moral philosophy, involves systematizing, defending, and recommending concepts of right and wrong. (*Internet Encyclopaedia of Philosophy*, 2007)

Such definitions are indeed true of our conduct in research. Unlike empirical research, literature-based research methodology does not require approval from an ethics committee, but it is not exempt from the codes of ethics. It is true that issues of confidentiality and consent do not apply to a literature-based methodology in the same way they do to empirical research because the data used in a literature-based methodology is already in the public domain. However, examples of literature that may *not* be in the public domain are hospital trust policies or papers. In this case, the researcher must seek the permission of relevant authors in relation to consent, anonymity and confidentiality.

In the following section we introduce you to a different dimension of ethics that is in keeping with the above definitions; that is, looking at ethics simply through the notion of rigour.

3.7.1 Understanding rigour as a dimension of ethics in research

In the context of research, rigour is defined in terms of a set of criteria against which the quality of the research is judged. These criteria are well elaborated in most research texts and are illustrated in Table 3.4.

However, these criteria, although very fitting in assessing the quality of any empirical research, cannot be applied in the same sense to comprehensive literature review methodology. Rather, three concepts used by the United Nations as part of the founding principle of public administration (Armstrong, 2005: 1), can be effectively applied to comprehensive literature reviews. These are:

Table 3.4 Rigour in quantitative and qualitative research (adapted from Lincoln and Guba, 1985)

Rigour in quantitative research	Rigour in qualitative research
Internal validity	Credibility
External validity	Transferability
Reliability	Dependability
Objectivity	Confirmability

1 **Integrity** – this refers to impartiality, fairness, honesty and truthfulness.
2 **Accountability** – this relates to your performance as a researcher. It involves the decisions that you will make about data collection and analysis and interpretation, all of which must stand scrutiny. It is also about how thorough you have been in critiquing, analyzing and interpreting the data.
3 **Transparency** – this refers to how accurate you have been in the conduct of your research; in other words, how true you have been to the methodology.

These concepts, as the United Nations uses them, are to 'ensure that public servants will put the interest of the public above their own' (Armstrong, 2005: 2). Similarly, research ought to seek that which will be in the interest of client care. These concepts can be translated to a framework for demonstrating rigour in research. They can be used to assess the quality of any empirical research and to demonstrate rigour in your comprehensive literature review. In Chapter 5, we will give a fuller discussion of the above principles of ethics as they apply to the comprehensive literature review methodology.

End-of-Chapter Learning Points

We hope that you have found this chapter helpful in understanding the tenets of literature-based methodology research design. The following are some of the key points highlighted in this chapter:

1 Literature-based research methodology involves researching work conducted and published by someone other than you. In other words, you are working with empirical research that was not designed by you.
2 Literature-based methodology needs to be designed in parallel with the process of primary research. It follows discrete steps in the design, thus making the research process, from identification of the research problem to reporting the research, transparent.
3 Two main types of literature review methodology are dealt with in this chapter: the systematic and comprehensive literature reviews. Each is informed by different philosophical perspectives. The comprehensive literature review should be informed by a combination of positivism and interpretivism.
4 There are four principles upon which the comprehensive literature review methodology is based. These are useful in guiding the design and the conduct of your research project.
5 Ethical considerations are important and are based on integrity, accountability and transparency in order to show rigour in your research project.

References

On research

Booth, A. (2001) 'Cochrane or cock-eyed? How should we conduct systematic reviews of qualitative research?', Paper presented at the Qualitative Evidence-Based Practice Conference, 14–16 May, Coventry University, Coventry, UK. www.leeds.ac.uk/educol/documents/00001724.htm (accessed 27 september 2011).

Brannen, J. (2005) 'Mixing methods: the entry of qualitative and quantitative approaches into the research process', International Journal of Social Research Methodology, 8(3), 173–184.

Carney, T.F. (1990) 'The ladder of analytical abstraction', cited in M.B. Miles and A.M. Huberman (eds) (1994) Qualitative Data Analysis (2nd edn). Thousand Oaks, CA: Sage.

Cooper, H. (2010) Research Meta-Synthesis and Meta-Analysis (4th edn). Los Angeles: Sage.

Crotty, M. (2003) The Foundations of Social Research: Meaning and Perspective in Social Research. London: Sage.

Denzin, N.K. and Lincoln, Y.S. (eds) (1998) Strategies of Qualitative Inquiry. Thousand Oaks, CA: Sage.

Higgins, P.J. and Green, S. (eds) (2011) The Cochrane Handbook for Systematic Review of Interventions: The Cochrane Collaboration. Chichestor: John Wiley & Sons Ltd.

Lincoln, Y.S. and Guba, E.G. (1985) Naturalistic Inquiry. Beverly Hills, CA: Sage.

Marshall, C. and Rossman, G.B. (1995) Designing Qualitative Research (2nd edn). Thousand Oaks, CA: Sage.

Merriam, S.B. (2001) Qualitative Research and Case Study Application in Education (2nd edn). San Francisco, CA: Jossey-Bass.

Mites, M.B. and Huberman, A.M. (eds) (1994) Qualitative Data Analysis (2nd edn). Thousand Oaks, CA: Sage.

Ndosi, M., Vinall, K., Hale, C., Bird, H. and Hill, J. (2011) 'The effectiveness of nurse-led care in people with rheumatoid arthritis: a systematic review', International Journal of Nursing Studies, 48(5), 642–654.

O'Brien, P.M.S. and Pipkin, F.B. (eds) (2007) Introduction to Research Methodology for Specialists and Trainees (2nd edn). London: RCOG Press.

Parahoo, K. (2006) Nursing Research: Principles, Process and Issues (2nd edn). Basingstoke: Palgrave Macmillan.

Paterson, B.L., Thorne, S.E., Canam, C. and Jillings, C. (2001) Meta-Study of Qualitative Health Research. Thousand Oaks, CA: Sage.

Polit, D.F. and Beck, C.T. (2006) Essentials of Nursing Research: Methods, Appraisal and Utilization (6th edn). Philadelphia, PA: Lippincott, Williams & Wilkins.

Randolph, J.J. (2009) 'A guide to writing the dissertation literature review', Practical Assessment, Research and Evaluation, 14(13), 1–13. www.pareonline.net/getvn.asp?v=14&n=13.

Sheldon, T.A. (2005) 'Making evidence synthesis more useful for management and policy-making', Health Service Research Policy, 10, Supplement 1, 1–15.

Streubert, H.L. and Carpenter, D.R. (2011) Qualitative Research in Nursing (5th edn). Philadelphia, PA: Wolters Kluwer/Lippincott, Williams & Wilkins.

Whittemore, R. and Knafl, K. (2005) 'The integrative review: updated methodology', Journal of Advanced Nursing, 52(5), 546–553.

On systematic and other literature review

Antman, E.M., Lau, J.M., Kulpenick, B., Mosteller, F. and Chalmers, T.C. (1992) 'A comparison of results of meta-analyses of randomized control trials and recommendations of clinical experts', *Journal of American Medical Association*, 268, 240–245.

Green, B.N., Johnson, C.D. and Adams, A. (2006) 'Writing a narrative literature review for peer-reviewed journal: secret of the trade', *Journal of Chiropractic Medicine*, 5(3), 101–117.

Hart, C. (1998) *Doing a Literature Review: Releasing the Social Science Research Imagination*. London: Sage.

Higgins, J.P.T. and Green, S. (eds) (2011) *Cochrane Handbook for Systematic Reviews of Interventions Version 5.1.0 [updated March 2011]*. The Cochrane Collaboration. Available at: www.cochrane-handbook.org.

Jesson, J., Matheson, L. and Lacey, F.M. (2011) *Doing Your Literature Review: Traditional and Systematic Reviews*. London: Sage.

Liberati, A., Altman, D., Tetxlaff, J., Mulrow, C., Gøtzsche, P., Larke, M., Devereaux, P., Kleijnen, J. and Moher, D. (2009) 'The PRISMA statement for reporting systematic reviews and meta-analyses of studies that evaluate health care interventions: explanation and elaboration', *Annals of Internal Medicine*, 151(4), W65–W94.

NHS Centre for Reviews and Dissemination (2009) *Systematic Reviews: CRD's Guidance for Undertaking Reviews in Health Care*. York: University of York. www.york.ac.uk/inst/crd/pdf/Systematic_Reviews.pdf (accessed 9 August 2011).

Oxman, A.D. (1994) 'Systematic reviews: checklist for review articles', *British Medical Journal*, 309, 648–661.

Petticrew, M. and Roberts, H. (2006) *Systematic Reviewing of Literature in the Social Sciences: A Practical Guide*. Oxford: Blackwell.

Popay, J. (ed.) (2006) *Moving Beyond Effectiveness in Evidence Synthesis: Methodological Issues in the Synthesis of Diverse Sources of Evidence*. London: National Institute for Health and Clinical Excellence (www.nice.org.uk).

Sackett, D.L., Richardson, W.S., Rosenberg, W.M.C. and Haynes, R.B. (1997) *Evidence-Based Medicine: How to Practice and Teach EBM*. London: Churchill Livingstone.

On policy and ethics

Armstrong, E.R. (2005) *Integrity, Transparency and Accountability in Public Administration: Recent Trends, Regional and International Developments and Emerging Issues*. Economic and Social Affairs, United Nations www.upan1.un.org/intradoc/groups/public/.../un/unpan020955.pdf.

Department of Health (2001) *Research Governance Framework for Health and Social Care*. London: Department of Health.

Internet Encyclopaedia of Philosophy (2007) 'Ethics'; *Encyclopaedia of Philosophy* [online] www.iep.utm.edu/e/ethics.htm.

Jarvis, P. (1997) *Ethics and Education for Adults in the Late Modern Society*. Leicester: National Institute of Adult and Continuing Education.

FOUR

Collecting Data by Searching and Sampling the Literature and Other Secondary Data Sources

| Aim and objectives |

The aim of this chapter is to focus on the process of searching for and sampling literature to use as data. By the end of this chapter you will be able to:

- Pinpoint the key words of your research question or statement
- Identify and select basic criteria to help you define the parameters of your search
- Recognize key sources you need to search
- Understand the difference between exploring the literature to define the scope of the project and searching the literature systematically to identify your data
- Appreciate how the structure of the sources and the structure of search software influence how you search
- Give a rationale for including or excluding literature found
- Recognize the importance of recording your search strategy and the details of items found
- Understand the options for recording details of items considered for your literature review.

4.1 Introduction

Look in any book on research methodology and you are likely to find statements like that made by Smith and Bird (2010: 53):

Discovering and reviewing what is already known is an essential exercise in the research process. It provides a context and starting point for your research, helps to define and direct your own approach and averts the dangers of potential plagiarism.

The search for material to consider in the preliminary review obviously needs to take place at the beginning of the research process. The search itself can inform you about your research problem and alert you to aspects of the topic you may not have considered. You will have begun a preliminary search when making a list of the studies relevant to your research on undertaking Student Activity 3.3 in Chapter 3.

The nature of your research will normally influence when the main search will take place. Sometimes the search is deliberately not undertaken until the empirical work has been completed: Punch (2005: 266) describes how the review will then 'be integrated into the research during the study, as in grounded theory'. He also states that there are several considerations to be made as to when to concentrate on the literature, such as the style of the research and the aims and objectives of the research study. Punch's points are clearly illustrated when undertaking research using the literature review methodology. Here, the literature is the source of the data for the research. Therefore, the searching has to be carried out before the data analysis can be undertaken.

Data may be found in places other than in literature. If 'the literature' is considered to be 'the written information about a subject' (Cambridge Dictionaries, 2011), it will be your main source of data, but it is possible that you can find data from non-print sources, such as a podcast where a researcher explains his/her findings or a PowerPoint presentation reviewing research or a conversation that you have with a researcher about his/her study.

As noted in Chapter 3, when discussing the literature review methodology, 'defining the sample' is not a linear but an iterative process. Similarly, Hart (2001: 24) suggests that this process 'might better be described as a helical process as you tend to go back and forth between sources following leads, expanding on previously acquired information and validating references'.

4.2 Identifying key words to use – why and how?

The first stage of literature searching is normally to define your topic and, in the literature review methodology, your research question/problem. Indeed, definition forms the first stage of the literature review methodology and, as such, has been considered in Chapter 2 (section 2.4.1). Currently, with some search tools, you can type in your research question and find some relevant literature. However, you are also likely to miss some key papers and find a fair amount of irrelevant material – irrelevant either because it does not focus on the subject of your literature review or because it is not the type of material you intend to include.

Not all search tools work like the search engines *Google* (www.google.co.uk) and *Yahoo! Search* (http://uk.search.yahoo.com). Software such as *Ovid* and *Ebsco*, which are used with databases such as *Cumulative Index to Nursing and Allied Health (CINAHL)*, usually search for what you type in as a phrase instead of searching for all the words you type in. So, for instance, although a search engine may find more than several million websites when you type in 'pain threshold level', *CINAHL* will find very few. However, if you identify the key words of your search, enter them separately and then combine the searches, you will retrieve better results: what you find is likely to include some articles that you would not find just using search engines.

Whichever way you choose to define your topic, it is possible that researchers may have used different terminologies, so it is important to identify all the key words that could be used to describe a subject. For instance, one author may refer to 'pressure sores', another to 'decubitus ulcers', a third to 'pressure ulcers' and a fourth to 'bedsores'. It is therefore useful to identify words related to your key words.

Additionally, some phrases are likely to be more significant than others for your search. Remember James, the senior nurse, who was particularly interested in changes in patients' body image in relation to stoma surgery from Chapter 1. If you are searching a database covering nursing journal articles, articles about body image relating to stoma surgery may not include the word 'patient' in the database record, although they will be about patients' body image. Therefore, you need to identify the really significant words. Moreover, it is important to note that some really significant words can also be rather general or vaguely defined. While 'home birth' is a term that is clearly defined, terms such as 'experiences' are open to different interpretations and are more likely to be described using alternative words, such as 'patient's perspective'.

Student Activity 4.1 will help you focus on the key words for your research topic.

■■■■■■■■■ **STUDENT ACTIVITY 4.1** ■■■■■■■■■

Look at the research question you wrote in Student Activity 2.6 in Chapter 2. If you do not have a note of what you wrote then, write it again.

Identify the significant words or phrases in your question and write them down. Create a table with a column for each significant word or phrase.

Think of all the *synonyms* (words or phrases that means exactly or nearly the same) and the *antonyms* (words or phrases meaning the opposite). Antonyms can be important. An article about incontinence, for example, may use the phrase continence care.

- If appropriate, look in nursing or medical dictionaries for formal names of conditions.
- Look in an English language thesaurus, e.g. the *Oxford Thesaurus of English* (Waite, 2009), for synonyms and antonyms of everyday words. List them under the relevant key words.

Keep your table as you will be returning to it later in the chapter.

Before moving on to the next section, it is worth considering PICO. PICO is a tool to help you identify significant key words and to help you ensure that your search covers all important aspects of your topic. It is designed mainly for questions related to *therapeutic interventions*. It stands for: population, intervention, comparison (or control or comparator) and outcome (Bettany-Saltikov, 2010). Student Example 4.1 shows how PICO can be applied to nursing and midwifery research.

Student Example 4.1 Using PICO

Consider Yvonne, the student midwife interested in researching the relationship between labour positions and outcome in terms of women's perineal health in Chapter 1.

Applying PICO, she would be looking for material that covered the following categories:

- Her *population* is women in labour
- Her *intervention* is a specific labour position
- Her *comparison* is other labour positions
- Her *outcome* is perineal health.

4.3 Identifying parameters for your search

The inclusion and exclusion criteria discussed in Chapter 3 need to be used to help you structure your search and limit the amount of information or data to a manageable number. Your definition of the research problem, if it has been sufficiently focused, will be your most important parameter. While a lot of information could be seen as being relevant and informative about your topic, it is easy to be side-tracked from your problem. Return to your research question or statement frequently and check that what you find is relevant to your purpose. However, before beginning to search you will find it helpful to clarify some limits for your search. Your research supervisor or module leader may offer some advice or guidelines. The following sections highlight some of the important parameters you need to consider.

4.3.1 What type of literature and other secondary data sources will you include and/or exclude – and why?

Some universities stipulate that a literature review should be based on journal articles, others on peer-reviewed journal articles. Of course, most published research appears in journals so that, if you are expected to focus on research, most of the literature you will cover will be journal articles.

If you decide to focus on (or to exclude) a particular type of literature or other data source, you should offer a rationale for doing this. For instance, if your search identifies a thesis that would be difficult for you to obtain but there is a journal article summarizing the findings, you could indicate that you are excluding theses because of the time and cost constraints of undertaking a comprehensive literature review for a student research project. If there has been a lot of research undertaken on your topic, you could indicate that you will only include studies with a clear methodology. Systematic reviews of randomized controlled trials are regarded as the gold standard of evidence-based healthcare but they may not always be available on or appropriate to the subject of your inquiry. As has been seen in Chapter 1, nursing-related topics frequently focus on qualitative evidence and systematic reviews of randomized controlled trials are usually quantitative. It is worth noting that Cleary-Holdforth and Leufer (2008) give details of a hierarchy of qualitative evidence. It is highly possible that you will need to include both qualitative and quantitative evidence.

If you are only including research journal articles in your review, it is often useful, when you are completing a preliminary search, to look at other materials, as they can give you a broad overview of your topic, helping you to scope and define your research problem. Books, including encyclopaedias, are especially useful for this.

4.3.2 Which dates will you include?

Generally, more recent material is more important than older material of a similar quality. Depending on its nature, newer material will build on and reflect what has already been published. Currency of information is more crucial with some subject areas than others. For example, in drug therapy, new treatments may be developed and contra-indications discovered, while changes in anatomy and physiology are likely to be rare. Additionally, some topics may have been the focus of attention for a year or two but may not have been featured recently, so that the bulk of your material will not be very recent. There will not always be a reason for this but if you know that new research was published in a particular year or that a significant conference took place on a topic/treatment that generated public controversy, you would expect to find more articles about that topic during that year and the following years.

Quite often you will find that all the literature you read about your research problem will refer back to a seminal paper, which may be quite old. You will need to decide whether to obtain a copy of the seminal paper and cite it directly or to include only papers that cite it.

4.3.3 Will you include material published in or published about particular parts of the world?

Your research problem or topic may be related to an aspect of nursing unique to the United Kingdom (UK) or possibly even unique to one of the UK countries. For instance, you may want to investigate the impact of Macmillan nurses. Macmillan nurses are funded by a British charity and are unique to the UK. All the literature referring to Macmillan nurses will be about nurses working in the UK. You may need to have done some searching to help you decide whether you will have to limit your review in this way. However, you will find that limiting your search by country can be difficult. When you look at brief details of articles as you search, it is not always easy to tell to which country they relate. Also, limiting your search to journals published in a certain country may mean that you will miss some articles relating to the country that were published elsewhere.

4.3.4 Will you limit your search to particular languages?

For the majority of research problems or topics you are tackling, it is likely that very little literature you identify will be in languages other than English. The National Library of Medicine website lists over 50 languages that are, or have been, represented in *Medline*, the huge database covering more than 5,500 current biomedical journals from the USA and over 80 other countries. Searching for records containing the phrase 'pressure ulcer', published from 1996 to November 2011, just over 15% of the articles are in languages other than English. However, when searching for records on *Medline* containing the phrases 'Macmillan nurse' or 'Macmillan nurses' or 'Macmillan nursing', all the articles identified are, unsurprisingly, in English. It is possible to obtain articles in foreign languages, though some expense may be involved. If a report or study that is particularly relevant and significant to your research is only available in a language other than English, you would be advised to discuss with your research supervisor whether to obtain a copy and whether to include it in your literature review. Obviously you cannot include anything in your review unless you have actually read it. If there is an English abstract that gives sufficient information about the item, you could consider using the abstract, but you would need to indicate that you had not read the original article. Obtaining translations of the articles can be difficult and expensive, so it is probably better to restrict your search to articles in English where possible.

4.3.5 Age and gender

With some research problems or topics, patients or populations, age and gender may not be relevant. In other cases, it may be defined by the research problem or topic itself, for example, if you are looking at infant feeding or adolescent pregnancy. However, you may choose to limit your study to a particular age group for a number of reasons: you may be working with a particular age group or gender, perhaps, or the amount of literature covering your research problem generally may be extremely large. For example, you may be particularly interested in the differences between adolescent diabetic patients' compliance in taking their prescribed drugs and that of adult patients. Similarly, you may be interested to examine the differences between men's and women's compliance.

4.4 Identifying sources for your data

The resources you use will depend mainly on three factors: the disciplines you have decided to include; the sources to which you have access; and the sources for different types of literature that you will be including. We will discuss these factors one at a time in the following sections.

4.4.1 Disciplines relevant to your research problem or topic

While nursing and midwifery have a rich body of literature, some research problems or topics may also touch on the literature of other disciplines. For instance, James's study of changes in body image in patients who had a stoma clearly touches on psychology. Examining the concept of body image in an article entitled 'Body image and the breast: the psychological wound', Chan (2010: 133) traces how 'a biophysical approach … linking its neurological, psychological and socio-cultural elements' was introduced to the study of body image. Although focusing on nursing and midwifery can easily be defended if you are undertaking a nursing or midwifery-related course of study, it may be that there is some extremely significant material which has appeared in the literature of related disciplines. You will need to decide whether or not to include it in your review. In these circumstances, the most important point to make is that you should justify your decision when writing your review.

4.4.2 Sources to which you have access

Some databases and journal articles are freely available on the internet, as are many reports and a vast amount of information on web pages. However, access to a lot of important sources has to be purchased and library services will usually do this for their registered users. You will need to check which sources your library services make available by looking on their website or referring to relevant guides or talking with the library staff.

4.4.3 Sources for different types of literature

There are two types of literature that are likely to be most useful for your research project: books and journal articles. The key places to look for these are discussed below.

4.4.3.1 Where to search for books

Library catalogues are excellent sources of information to help you identify relevant books. However, they do usually also cover types of material other than books, such as theses, DVDs and CDs. Some even include details of journal articles, though most will only indicate the journal titles which the library holds. University libraries are likely to purchase material relevant to the course of study you are undertaking and library services provided by employers are likely to purchase material relevant to your employment.

The catalogues of relevant specialist collections are very often freely available on the internet and are often worth searching, even if you cannot borrow materials from the library. If you identify material on them which is not available locally, you will need to decide if the content is likely to warrant the cost or effort of obtaining or viewing the item, either by requesting to borrow it through your library's interlibrary loan service or by negotiating to visit a library that holds it. The Royal College of Nursing Library is a good example of a specialist collection. The RCN Library (www.rcn.org.uk/library) aims to purchase and archive all nursing-related books published in the UK. English language books from other countries are also added to their stock. It includes good coverage of grey literature, 'a range of published and unpublished material which is not normally identifiable through conventional methods of bibliographic control' (Hart, 2001: 94), for example, leaflets and booklets published by organizations such as charities and information produced by the government. Additionally, it has an excellent and growing collection of British nursing theses. Where materials are available electronically, links are provided in the catalogue records.

WorldCat (www.worldcat.org) covers the collections of more than 10,000 libraries worldwide and, although not specific to nursing, it does include nursing materials in a variety of languages. *COPAC* (www.copac.ac.uk) covers over 66 national, academic and specialist libraries in the UK and Ireland. It is particularly useful as it includes the catalogue of the British Library, which by law must hold one copy of every book, pamphlet, journal and newspaper published in the UK.

4.4.3.2 Where to search for journal articles

There are four key places to look for journal articles: bibliographic databases, full-text databases, citation databases and internet search engines.

1   **Bibliographic databases** – Bibliographic databases do not always include the full text, though it is often possible to link to the full text of the article from the database record if your library has purchased access to the full text. Essential information to help searchers identify and find relevant material is selected from each journal article for inclusion on the database. Basic information about the article, including the author(s), article title, journal title, year of publication, volume, part/issue and pages is provided. You will find that databases vary in how they present this information. For instance, many will only give the author's surname and initials, not their full name, and some abbreviate the journal title. Where an abstract summarizing the article is available, this will help in deciding if the material is likely to be relevant to your research. Usually subject headings are assigned to each item. These are also known as indexing terms or descriptors and are usually assigned by information professionals with at least a broad knowledge of the subject area.

Some databases, notably the *Cumulative Index for Nursing and Allied Health* (*CINAHL*) include a lot more detail in their records, such as place of publication, author affiliation, the type of article and whether it is peer reviewed or not and, with research articles, the type of research instrument used.

The main databases covering nursing and midwifery literature are *CINAHL*, *British Nursing Index* (*BNI*) and *Maternity and Infant Care*, although *Medline* also has significant coverage of nursing literature.

(a) *CINAHL*

The number of journal articles covered by *CINAHL* will depend on which version your library service has purchased. The basic version covers more than 3,000 journals, but *CINAHLPlus* includes details of articles from over 4,600 journals. It is also possible to purchase the database with some full text, with over 600 journals for the basic version and over 770 journals for *CINAHLPlus*. In addition to journal articles, *CINAHL* includes details of some books, book chapters, theses, conference proceedings, standards of practice, educational software and audio-visual material. Most material is from the United States, although a significant number of UK journals are covered: when checked early in 2012, approximately 25% of the journal articles included were from journals published in the UK. It includes some material from as early as the 1930s but most records are more recent and the number of records being added annually continues to grow.

(b) *BNI* (*British Nursing Index*)

The *BNI* covers approximately 250 journals and focuses more on literature from UK journals, though it does cover other key English language titles. It also concentrates on nursing and midwifery, though it does select and include nursing and midwifery-related articles from some medical, allied health and health management journals. It includes references dating back to 1994.

(c) *Maternity and Infant Care*

Maternity and Infant Care includes references to articles from over 550 international English language journals, books, and grey literature relating to pregnancy, labour, birth, postnatal care and neonatal care and the first year of an infant's life. It is produced in the UK. The database was originally known as *Midirs* and it is still possible to subscribe to the *Midirs Reference Database* via the company *Midirs* (www.midirs.org).

(d) *Medline*

This database includes life sciences concentrating on biomedicine. It covers approximately 5,500 worldwide journals in 39 languages. According to the *National Library of Medicine Catalog* (National Center for Biotechnology Information, 2011), it currently covers 256 nursing and midwifery titles. Most material included is from 1946 to the present but it does include some older material.

It is worth using all of these sources, depending on your subject. Not only are some journal titles unique to each resource, but also their records are different. It can be useful for instance, to compare an abstract from *CINAHL* or *Medline* with the indexer-written abstract from *BNI*. Additionally, the indexing terms are different in each database and, although you will need to adapt your search to each database, you are likely to identify some unique records in each. For instance, Brazier and Begley (1996) found that only 20% of their search results appeared in both *Medline* and *CINAHL*.

Other bibliographic databases are listed in Table 4.1.

Table 4.1 Other bibliographic databases

Types of database	Usage
AMED	For material about professions allied to medicine, complementary therapy and palliative care
The Cochrane Library	For high-quality, independent evidence to inform healthcare decision-making, including systematic reviews of healthcare interventions
Embase	For coverage of pharmaceutical and allied health literature, with a European focus
Health Management Information Consortium (HMIC)	For health management and health care policy
PsycINFO	For behavioural sciences material

2 **Full-text databases** – Publishers and companies who make journals available electronically also provide basic search facilities in most instances so that you can search across the journals to which they provide access. Publishers often allow anyone to search journals on their websites. However, although some do make a certain amount of material freely accessible, most will only allow access to people registered with an organization that has purchased access.

3 **Citation databases** – Citation indexes serve two main purposes. They will allow you to see how frequently an author has been cited. Scullion and Guest (2007: 116) warn that 'care should be taken when doing this as there are many reasons why an author may cite an article and not necessarily because it is significant to their subject'. Frequently cited authors are likely to be important authors, but they could also be cited because they are notorious. Secondly, citation indexes can lead you to relevant journal articles because they cite significant articles which you have already identified. Although you can track back to significant material by looking at the references cited by an author, citation indexes allow you to track forwards from an article. As yet the nursing literature is not particularly well represented in the key citation indexes. The *ISI Web of Science*, which includes the *Science Citation Index* and the *Social Sciences Citation Index* does include some coverage of nursing materials, but generally the coverage is relatively low compared with medicine. Courtney and Jones (2006: 6) noted that:

...of the 1712 scientific journals listed in Social Science Edition database of ISI, only 32 journals are ranked under the nursing category. Similarly, in the Science Edition database, of the 5120 journals ranked only 33 appear under the nursing category.

In 2012 nursing coverage has increased a little: 87 nursing journals are covered in *Social Sciences Citation Index* and 89 in *Science Citation Index*. Some bibliographic databases, for instance *SciVerse Scopus, Medline* and, significantly, *CINAHL*, do add details of articles cited with each reference and provide a facility to search them.

4 **Internet search engines** – The internet is huge and growing – a resource of millions of interlinked websites, including links to millions of journal articles, documents, images,

videos, maps and other materials. However, not all documents are freely available on the internet, and not all information available on the internet is reliable. Journal articles and books usually indicate something about the credentials of the authors but many people have pointed out that there is no control over material placed on the internet: 'The problem with the internet is that anyone can put anything on it with no kind of censorship or quality control, so you may be finding sites that contain information that is inappropriate, incorrect or even harmful' (Freeman and Thompson, 2009: 93). It is worth noting sites recommended by expert colleagues or contacts. It is also important to note sites that are recommended on your university site and on other sites that you trust. However, you will not find all you need on these sites and will often need to make use of search engines: '…software which searches the Internet looking for web pages which match the terms you have typed into the search box' (Freeman and Thompson, 2009: 92). It is important to note that they do not usually cover the contents of databases such as *BNI* and *CINAHL* or library catalogues. However, increasingly, library services which have purchased access to electronic journals and books are enabling their members to access material direct from search engines rather than logging on to the library web page.

At the end of 2011, Phil Bradley detailed over 170 search engines on his website 'Making the Net a Lot Easier' (www.philb.com). He commented about *Google* (www.google.co.uk) that it 'is always a good bet, since it has the largest index' (Bradley, 2011). There are search engines intended to retrieve high-quality information, notably journal articles, and these are designed for use by academics and students. Of these, *Google Scholar* is the one which is most mentioned in nursing literature, though *Scirus* is occasionally included. It is worth getting to know two or three search engines well, as you will sometimes find different sites by using different search engines and sites may be presented in a different order.

STUDENT ACTIVITY 4.2

Look at the table you have devised from Student Activity 4.1. List the disciplines that you could draw on in your search.

Decide whether you are going to set parameters for your search and, if so, what they will be. Create another chart, giving:

- the nature of the parameter, e.g. type of material
- the detail of the parameter, e.g. peer-reviewed research journal articles
- your rationale for setting the parameter, e.g. university guideline.

Identify and list the sources you will consider using for your search by looking at the websites of library services to which you have access. Also look at any guides produced by your library services or university and talk with library staff. Remember to look for resources to help you find evidence from the related disciplines you have identified as well as looking for resources relevant to nursing and midwifery.

Discuss your parameters and your sources with your research supervisor.

4.5 Searching

Generally, all the search tools you will be using will be different from each other and it will be worth your while getting to know how they work. Some library services make available a tool, sometimes known as a single-search, cross-search or federated search tool, which allows you to search across several resources at once, such as:

- Your university library catalogue
- Internet search engines, including *Google*, *YouTube*
- Bibliographic databases, for example *CINAHL*, *BNI* or *Medline*
- Full-text databases.

Also, databases purchased from the same company can usually be searched together. It may be worth searching across several tools at once when you are starting out and wanting to define the scope of your research project. It can be helpful in indicating which tools are likely to be the most useful for you.

Your search will need to be 'systematic and explicit', as recommended by Auston, Cahn and Selden (1992), as the tools will be structured differently because their records include variable information. Although different search software programs may work in similar ways to each other, there are often also some differences. It is better to search one tool at a time when you are carrying out the search for data related to your research problem/topic. Most university libraries offer tuition and may also produce guides to using the tools they make available or provide links to guides available on the internet. Luckily, there are some common traits to the different types of tool.

4.5.1 Searching bibliographic databases

In this section, we will examine both basic and advanced searching of bibliographic databases. It is important to understand that your search may be affected by both:

- the structure of the database, including the detail in each record (e.g. the databases *CINAHL*, *BNI* or *Medline*); and
- the software used for searching the database (e.g. *Ovid*, *Ebsco* or *ProQuest*)

4.5.1.1 Basic searching of bibliographic databases

As noted in section 4.2 'Identifying key words to use – why and how?', the software used with most bibliographic databases searches for the words that you type in as a phrase. Most searching software available at present searches for exactly what you type in. It is unlikely that you will find many records of journal articles containing the title of your research project. It is usually better to search on your keywords, combining with the word '*and*'. For instance, if you just type in 'changes in patients' body image in relation to stoma surgery' you are unlikely to find any material. However, if you type in 'stoma and body image' you will retrieve some relevant references. You could add in other words, such as 'change', but the more that you add in using '*and*', the less you will find. Most software will allow you to combine search words once you have entered them. This will allow you to try different combinations of words without having to type them in again.

The term '*and*' is known as a Boolean operator (after the mathematician Georges Boole). The other most useful Boolean operator is '*or*'. Using '*and*' will find both terms it joins, but using '*or*' will find either of the terms. It is very useful in structuring searches when there are several synonyms for a term: you can create clusters of terms for your concepts using '*or*'. For example, you can search for 'stoma or colostomy or ileostomy', then search for 'body image or self concept', then you can combine the two clusters using '*and*'.

The fact that most bibliographic database software searches for exactly what you type in has other implications. It will not usually correct your spelling or ask you 'did you really mean....?' If you do not find any records with your search term when you think there should be some results, start by checking your spelling. Another point to consider: if you search on the keyword 'paediatrics', you will not retrieve records where the American spelling, 'pediatrics' is used; you will also not retrieve records with just 'paediatric' – without the final 's'. Most software offers two tools to help with this. A truncation symbol, often an asterisk (*) or dollar sign ($), can be used at the end of a word to retrieve all words with the same stem. For example, paediatric* will retrieve 'paediatric' and 'paediatrics' – and also 'paediatrician' and 'paediatricians'. The other tool is the wildcard, usually a question mark (?). For example, searching for 'p?ediatric' will find both 'paediatric' and 'pediatric'. The wildcard will find a letter or no letter, so that 'wom?n' will find 'woman' and 'women'. What it does not usually find are the same words with and without a hyphen, such as 'premenstrual' and 'pre-menstrual' – you would need to search for these separately.

STUDENT ACTIVITY 4.3

Look back at the list of sources you created in Student Activity 4.2 in this chapter.

Log on to the bibliographic databases you listed and look for the help information they offer about searching. Alternatively, check any guides to databases offered by your library.

Identify the following:

- How to combine different search terms with 'and' and with 'or'
- Other Boolean operators which might be useful

(Continued)

(Continued)

- What the truncation symbol is
- What the wildcard is.

N.B. You need only do this once for all the databases using the same software. For example, if *CINAHL* and *Medline* are both on your list and are both made available to you with Ebsco software, you do not need to repeat the exercise for both databases.

4.5.1.2 Advanced searching of bibliographic databases

Probably the most significant information added to the records of bibliographic databases is the subject headings, sometimes called indexing terms, descriptors or controlled vocabulary. The database will have a set of headings from which the indexers select to describe the material. It is worth remembering that most headings used in *CINAHL* and *Medline* are based on American usage and those used in *BNI* are British. Due to their nursing focus, *CINAHL* and *BNI* have a higher proportion of specialist nursing headings compared with *Medline*, which concentrates more on medical literature. For example, *BNI* uses the heading 'health visiting', where *CINAHL* and *Medline* use 'community health nursing'. *CINAHL* also offers 'community mental health nursing', which does not appear in the *Medline* thesaurus – *BNI* uses 'community psychiatric nursing' for this.

Often these headings are structured in a thesaurus so that you can see them in the context of broader and narrower headings, as in the following example, based on *CINAHL*. Underneath the heading 'labor', the heading 'labor stages' is given; and underneath 'labor stages' are specific labour stages (Figure 4.1).

Using the subject headings can be useful in your search and may save you some time. For example, *CINAHL* uses the heading 'birthing positions' for material about 'the position the mother is in for delivery' (*CINAHL* scope note). You may have written down some synonyms and related words, such as 'labour positions', 'birth positions', 'squatting', 'supine', 'semi-sitting' and 'birthing seat'. An author may use any or all of these in the article title and they may appear in the abstract, but the heading selected for the article will be 'birthing positions'. Most searching software allows you to 'map' from a word to the heading that is used within that particular database.

Knowing which heading a particular database uses for your topic can help you find a lot of relevant material quickly. However, databases vary in the detail of their indexing. For instance, in *BNI* no more than four headings are assigned to each article. In *CINAHL* and *Medline*, numerous headings can be applied and sub-headings are also used to allow for greater precision. Examples for sub-headings that can be used with 'birthing positions' on *CINAHL* include 'adverse effects', 'trends' and 'evaluation'. Additionally, *CINAHL* and *Medline* also assign headings

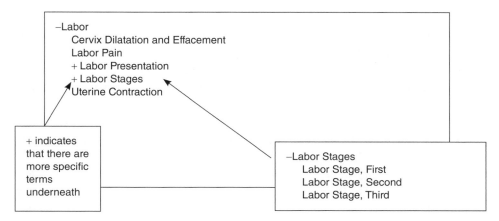

Figure 4.1 Example of headings in context in a bibliographic database thesaurus, based on *CINAHL* (including American spellings)

as major or minor headings. If a topic is a major feature of a journal article, the relevant heading will appear as a major heading; if it is of lesser importance, it will be a minor heading. For instance, in *CINAHL*, the article 'Women's positions during the second stage of labour: views of primary care midwives' (De Jonge et al., 2008) is assigned the major headings 'birthing positions', 'labour stage, second' and 'midwives'. Minor headings are 'adult', 'attitude of health personnel – evaluation', 'audio-recording', 'consent', 'decision making', 'patient', 'empirical research', 'female', 'field notes', 'focus groups', 'middle age', 'Netherlands', 'pregnancy', 'purposive sample', 'thematic analysis' and 'human'. In *BNI*, the headings used for the same article are 'labour', 'patients: positioning', 'midwife patient relations' and 'maternity rights'.

Do not rely totally on the headings as you may be able to see relevance in an article where the indexer does not select the heading you think appropriate. For example, a thesis entitled 'The labour position trial: a randomized, controlled trial of hands and knees positioning for women labouring with a foetus in occipito-posterior position' (Stremler, 2003) is included on *CINAHL* but is not indexed with the heading 'birthing positions'. The major headings assigned are 'patient positioning' and 'labor' (spelt in the American style). Additionally, on databases which assign a smaller number of headings to each record, a key feature of the article may not be indexed. Therefore, it is good practice also to search for your key words in other parts of the record. In fact, many people undertaking systematic reviews will go to the trouble of hand searching significant journals, looking through the contents pages to identify relevant articles as well as using the databases. However, it is unlikely that you will need to do this for your research project.

4.5.1.3   Refining your search of bibliographic databases

You can use the structure of the record and the database to help you with your search. Most databases default to searching for your key word in any of the title, abstract, subject heading and author fields or sections of the record. If you are finding too many irrelevant records with your key word or key words, you can restrict your search to find articles with your search word in a specific part of the record. For instance, articles with your search word in the title are more likely to be relevant than an article with your search word in the abstract but not in the title. Also, if you are searching for the headings on *CINAHL* and *Medline*, you can restrict your search to articles where the heading is a major heading, so that the topic is likely to be central to the article.

Many databases will include 'limiters' in the records. *CINAHL* includes, for instance, details of date of publication, age groups, publication type, language, and, in journal subset, place of publication. You can use these limiters. Most databases will allow you to limit the date of the publications you find, so that you only find the most recent material. You can also search for material from a particular year or years. With *CINAHL*, you can restrict your search to peer-reviewed articles and, using the 'publication type' limit, to research papers. The 'publication type' limits relating to research on *Medline* are much more specific, for example, clinical trials and comparative studies. With *BNI*, there is not a limit for peer review or for document type. However, the indexers will include the word 'research' in the abstract if the article is reporting research, so by including the word 'research' as one of your key words in a search on *BNI*, you will retrieve research articles. Filters are likely to be used by people undertaking a review of all the randomized controlled trials on a topic, in order to produce guidelines for practice.

People who are very concerned to ensure they find all studies of a particular design often use search filters: 'collections of search terms designed to retrieve selections of records' (Glanville, 2008: 6). Filters are likely to be used by people undertaking a review of all the randomized controlled trials on a topic, in order to produce guidelines for practice.

Student Example 4.2   Limiting a search to UK material

After reading Student Example 1.4 in Chapter 1, Tom was interested to find out how nurses were using personal digital assistants (PDAs) in the UK. Checking to see whether he was likely to find much, he searched on *CINAHL*, searching for articles that reported practice in the UK. He used the subject headings for the UK and also searched for articles published in the UK, using the *journal subset* limit. Limiting his search to the years 2010–2011, he found only two articles that could have been about UK practice. One had been in a journal published in the UK, with an author based in Cardiff. However, the abstract indicated that the article

---

was not specific to the UK – and the article was about trainee doctors. The other, in a nursing journal published in the USA, by a team from a British hospital, only mentioned PDAs in passing, describing how patients were asked to use them in a research project. He concluded that the use of PDAs in the UK was so new that not much had yet been written about it.

If you are finding too little literature, you can try using more synonyms or related words to broaden your search. You can also use the structure of the thesaurus to help you broaden the search. For instance, if you are looking for articles about lung diseases, you can include specific lung diseases. Alternatively, when searching using the subject headings on databases such as *CINAHL* and *Medline*, there is a facility, known as exploding, which allows you to search on a heading with all its narrower headings in one go. If you use this, in this example, it will include all the specific lung diseases.

4.5.2 Searching full-text databases

Library services often purchase access to a number of electronic journals from one supplier for their readers and the search facilities made available by the supplier or publisher can be used. Usually an abstract will be provided if one is published with the article in the journal but rarely are any indexing terms assigned. Searching full-text databases can be useful for items you are unable to find using bibliographic databases. Something may be mentioned in the full text of an article which is not significant enough to feature in the record on a bibliographic database and hence does not appear in the article title or abstract and is not reflected in the headings. Also, some journals may be included in full-text databases which are not covered by the bibliographic databases.

You may not be able to complete as sophisticated a search as you could on a bibliographic database. If you search for your key words in the full text of articles, you may well find many articles that only mention your search word in passing. It is usually possible to look for search words in the titles of articles or in the abstracts and it is usually possible to use the Boolean operators.

4.5.3 Searching citation databases

If you have found a paper or an author extremely relevant to your study, it can sometimes be useful to use citation databases, like the *ISI Web of Science*, to find other authors who have cited the paper or the author. To do this, you will need to select the *Cited reference search* option on the citation database. Be aware that the same papers may be cited differently by different authors. For instance, the title of Hayward's 1975 study *Information – A Prescription against Pain* is sometimes not given and the work is referred to as *Study in Nursing Care* or *Royal College of Nursing Study in Nursing Care*. It is a good idea to try different combinations of the details of the paper, e.g. the author's surname, the year of the paper and the journal title. Citation search facilities available on bibliographic databases sometimes work in a different way. On *Medline*, for instance, you will need to find a paper first: you can then select to see the details of the articles which have cited the journal. On *CINAHL*, the citation search facility is not found alongside the keyword searches but can be found under the *more* tab. Don't forget that citation searching is likely to be more productive with papers which are not very recent as there will not have been time for articles to have been written and published citing a recent paper.

4.5.4 Searching the internet

Search engines use software which automatically searches for and adds information about the resources it finds to the information covered by that search engine. There is generally no human input into the process, no indexing terms added and no abstracting undertaken.

Search engines will generally search for all the terms you type in separately, not as a phrase. For example, if you type in 'prevention and detection of bowel cancer', the search engine will look for the words 'prevention', 'detection', 'bowel' and 'cancer'. However, Karen Blakeman has noted in her blog, that *Google* is changing – '...now, if it cannot find all your search words, it will ignore some of them' – and it is increasingly collecting search and personal information about you, which can influence your search results, and not always for the better (Blakeman, 2012).

There are some tips that you can use to try to enhance your chances of retrieving relevant information:

- With some search engines it is possible to use a UK version. Some, like *Google*, will automatically take you to the UK version. Others, like *Bing* (www.bing.com), offer you the opportunity to search for pages only from the UK or to narrow your results so that you see only pages from the UK. Be wary as you will still retrieve links to some non-UK material.
- If you want to search for a phrase, put double inverted commas around the words, such as "community nurses", otherwise you will find that you retrieve some websites that mention 'community' and 'nurses' but not 'community nurses'.
- Look for an advanced search facility. Where this is present, it will usually offer you a lot more search facilities.
- After searching, check to see what has actually been searched. If you have searched 'community nurses' it may tell you that it has actually searched 'community nursing' and ask you if you really wanted 'community nurses'.

4.5.5 Some important things to do while you search

You will need to check back to your research question from Student Activity 2.7 in Chapter 2 and your chart of concepts and your parameters from Student Activities 4.1 and 4.2 earlier in this chapter to ensure that the information you find is relevant and fits your criteria. If you cannot find enough relevant information you may need to reconsider your topic or your parameters. It is a good idea to keep a record of your search strategy and your references as you go along: you will need to report on your strategy when you write up research and will need to give details of your references. Check if your university offers any guidelines for writing up the search strategy in your dissertation – or ask your research supervisor. It is likely that the main things you will need to include will be details of the parameters and sources you selected. Be sure to provide a rationale for your choices. You may also need to indicate the search strategy you used for each of your sources. Most databases will allow you to print out your search strategy, often called the search history; this could be added in an appendix. Alternatively, you could create a chart showing the key words you used in each database, indicating which of these were subject headings and showing how the key words were combined, along with the numbers of hits.

Student Example 4.3   Important things to do while you search

While Tom, from Student Example 4.2, searched for information about the use of the personal digital assistants in the UK, he frequently checked back to the research question he had written and to his chart of concepts and his parameters. He did this to ensure that the information he found fitted the criteria he had chosen. However, he could not find enough information that was relevant within the parameters he had set. He consulted an Information Specialist in the library to check that he was searching efficiently, taking with him details of his search strategies (having printed out the search history from each of the databases he used). He concluded that his search strategy was robust and that little was yet written about the use of these devices in the UK. He decided he would need to reconsider his research question or his parameters and made an appointment to discuss this with his research supervisor. It was agreed that he should broaden his focus beyond use of the devices in the UK. Luckily he had kept a record of the relevant references he had seen that were not about UK practice, using the Referencing tab on *Microsoft Word*.

His research supervisor advised him that using reference management software would be a good idea as not only would it help him keep track of his references and lay them out in the format required more easily, it would also be possible to download references straight from the databases to the reference management software as he searched. His supervisor mentioned that there were several reference management programmes freely available on the internet but particularly recommended the software made available by the university. Tom made a note to check for information about the software offered by the university on its website or to ask in the library.

End-of-Chapter Learning Points

We hope you have had time to reflect on what you have learnt from the student activities. The following are some of the key points highlighted in this chapter:

1 You will have realized that searching can be time consuming. You need to allow yourself sufficient time to undertake your search but you will also need to be realistic and decide on the amount of time you can afford to spend searching.
2 Taking time to plan your search and to understand how your search tools work can save you time in the long run.
3 You may need to compromise on the number of tools you search and if, early on, you are not finding sufficient usable data, you should consider whether you need to broaden your research topic or consider a different angle. It is vital that you discuss your progress with your research supervisor. If you are finding too much data, you may need to reduce the number of search tools you use or add additional parameters.
4 Not all search tools work like *Google* and not everything is available via *Google*.
5 Not everything is available full text electronically.
6 You need to provide a rationale for your searching strategies and decisions when writing up your research findings.

References

Auston, I., Cahn, M.A. and Selden, C.R. (1992) *Literature Search Methods for the Development of Clinical Practice Guidelines*. Prepared for the Agency for Health Care Policy and Research, Office of the Forum for Quality and Effectiveness in Health Care, Forum Methodology Conference, 13–16, December. Available at: www.nlm.nih.gov/nichsr/litsrch.html (accessed 29/11/11).

Bettany-Saltikov, J. (2010) 'Learning how to undertake a systematic literature review: part 1', *Nursing Standard*, 24(50): 47–55.

Blakeman, K. (2012) *Karen Blakeman's Blog*, www.rba.co.uk/wordpress (accessed 09/02/12).

Bradley, P. (2011) *Making the Net Easier: Which Search Engine When?*, www.philb.com/whichengine.htm (accessed 01/02/12).

Brazier, H. and Begley, C.M. (1996) 'Selecting a database for literature searches in nursing: MEDLINE or CINAHL?', *Journal of Advanced Nursing*, 24(4), 868–875.

Cambridge Dictionaries (2011) *Cambridge Learner's Dictionary*. Cambridge: Cambridge University Press. Available at: www.dictionary.cambridge.org/dictionary/learner-english (accessed 19/03/12).

Chan, L. (2010) 'Body image and the breast: the psychological wound', *Journal of Wound Care*, 19(4), 133–138.

Cleary-Holdforth, J. and Leufer, T. (2008) 'Essential elements in developing evidence-based practice', *Nursing Standard*, 23(2), 42–46.

Courtney, M. and Jones, J. (2006) 'Impact fever: what is it all about?', *Australian Journal of Advanced Nursing*, 23(4), 6–7.

De Jonge, A., Teunissen, D.A.M. van Diem, M.Th., Scheepers, P.L.H. and Lagro-Janssen, A.L.M. (2008) 'Women's positions during the second stage of labour: views of primary care midwives', *Journal of Advanced Nursing* , 63(4), 347–356.

Freeman, B. and Thompson, D. (2009) *Fundamental Aspects of Finding and Using Information: A Guide for Students of Nursing and Health.* London: Quay Books.

Glanville, J. (2008) 'Searching shortcuts: finding and appraising search filters', *He@lth Information on the Internet*, 63, 6–8.

Hart, C. (2001) *Doing a Literature Search: A Comprehensive Guide for the Social Sciences.* London: Sage.

Hayward, J. (1975) *Information – A Prescription against Pain.* London: Royal College of Nursing.

National Center for Biotechnology Information (2011) *National Library of Medicine Catalog,* www.ncbi.nlm.nih.gov/nlmcatalog (accessed 19/03/12).

Punch, K.F. (2005) *Introduction to Social Research: Quantitative and Qualitative Approaches* (2nd edn). London: Sage.

Scullion, P.A. and Guest, D.A. (2007) *Study Skills for Nursing and Midwifery Students.* Maidenhead: Open University Press.

Smith, S. and Bird, D. (2010) 'What do we know already? Searching the literature', in P. Roberts and H. Priest (eds), *Healthcare Research: A Textbook for Students and Practitioners.* Chichester: John Wiley.

Stremler, R.L. (2003) 'The labour position trial: a randomized, controlled trial of hands and knees positioning for women labouring with a fetus in occipitoposterior position', PhD dissertation, University of Toronto, Toronto. (cited in *CINAHL*).

Waite, M. (ed.) (2009) *Oxford Thesaurus of English* (3rd edn). Oxford: Oxford University Press.

Websites

www.google.co.uk
www.rcn.org.uk/library
http://uk.search.yahoo.com
www.worldcat.org
www.copac.ac.uk
www.midirs.org
www.philb.com
www.bing.com

FIVE

Ethical Considerations when Critiquing Literature-Based Data

| Aim and objectives |

The aim of this chapter is to explore issues of ethics and to consider their implications for the comprehensive literature review research methodology. By the end of this chapter you will be able to:

- Demonstrate knowledge of the general principles of ethics in research
- Understand the application of the three ethical principles underpinning comprehensive literature review methodology
- Apply the principles of ethics in setting evaluative criteria for data analysis of the selected literature.

5.1 Introduction

Research evidence plays a key role in clinical decisions regarding client care. As you have seen in Chapter 3, it is imperative that you have a sound knowledge of ethics related to research so that it can be applied effectively to the review of literature. The key point to remember is that the findings of the studies you will be critiquing are the raw data (The Economics & Social Research Council, 2011). Essentially, ethics is about ensuring proper research conduct. In other words, researchers are expected to adhere to honest research practices. It asks the researcher the simple question of what is acceptable and what is not; ethics is about ensuring that research is conducted to a high quality (Department of Health, 2001; Davenport, 2010).

Sometimes research can be abused as ethical misconduct can misrepresent evidence and thus seriously impact upon clinical decisions on client care. In addition, comprehensive literature reviews pose a particular challenge in so far as they have been criticized for lacking a systematic process. Consequently, these research findings may be seen to have little contribution to make to the evidence that informs policy and clinical decisions. This leads us to consider two important aspects:

1   The ethical conduct of the researcher using data from a secondary source in the literature review research methodology
2   The extent to which the primary researchers of the papers that you are critiquing have demonstrated ethical conduct in their research.

Research ethics refers to the moral principles cited by Beauchamp and Childress (2008) – beneficence and non-maleficence, justice and autonomy – that guide research from its inception through to completion and publication of results and beyond. It is also about avoiding error, protecting against falsification or misrepresenting data and ensuring that researchers can be held accountable to the public (Resnik, 2011). In this chapter we consider the applicability of the principles of ethics to the literature review methodology. The three concepts of integrity, transparency and accountability (introduced in Chapter 3) are further explored.

5.2 Integrity, transparency and accountability

It is important to remember that without ethically thought-out criteria there is little against which you can make judgement and interpretation when critiquing the literature. We will take you through the three concepts upon which to base your evaluation of the literature. This will serve as a guide to understanding the relevance of ethics in the literature review methodology. This is illustrated in Figure 5.1.

In most research texts, writing about the evaluation of the quality of research refers to integrity as the overarching criterion encompassing both transparency and accountability. While acknowledging that these three criteria have overlapping characteristics, our position is that in comprehensive literature review methodology the need for explicit distinction of integrity, transparency and accountability is crucial. There are differences between them that are fundamental to the development of evaluative criteria for critiquing literature. A comprehensive literature review methodology raises ethical considerations that are different from those of empirical research. In the following sections, the three criteria for judging quality and evaluating rigour will be examined more closely. For the meantime, consider the following student activity, which asks you to question your own basic ethical principles.

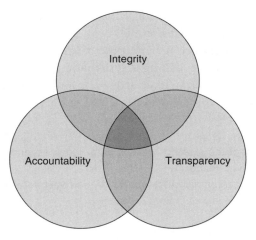

Figure 5.1 A conceptual framework for understanding the applicability of ethics: a pluralistic approach (adapted from Armstrong, 2005)

━━━━━━━━ **STUDENT ACTIVITY 5.1** ━━━━━━━━

Choose one research paper you have selected for your research project and consider the following questions posed by *The Research Ethics Guidebook* (Economic & Social Research Council, 2011: 1) for researchers using the literature review methodology:

- How will you review the chosen piece of research accurately and fairly?
- Do the data you are reviewing raise ethical questions that need addressing?
- If the reviewer (you) needs further information from the researcher, would you contact the researcher for more details?
- If you ask the study author for more details, how will you ensure that any exchange respects ethical principles? For example, will it affect the confidentiality originally promised to study participants?

In this exercise, you may not be able to provide a comprehensive answer to the questions above, but they are definitely food for thought for the future. Bring these up at your action learning sets and discuss these with other students.

However, there is one vital question that you must always bear in mind when using other people's research findings: *What are your obligations as a researcher using literature-based data?* While the potential for harm in a comprehensive literature review (as in all literature-based methodology) may not be as significant as in empirical research, we invite you to consider the harm that may result when the principles of ethics are not properly addressed.

Compare your findings with another student and share these with other students in your action learning set.

5.2.1 The ethical principle of integrity

Figure 5.2 shows the three key principles that define integrity. They are *honesty*, *truthfulness* and *fairness*. It is important that you (the researcher) strive not to

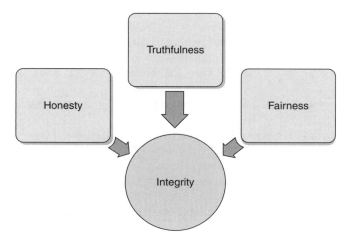

Figure 5.2 The three principles of integrity (adapted from Armstrong, 2005)

fall short of these principles when dealing with the processes of collecting, ana-lyzing and interpreting data, along with reporting the findings of your research.

There are a number of issues that need to be considered in order to ensure *hon-esty* in research. These can be summarized as follows:

- Declaring your own biases and personal ambitions so as to ensure objectivity in posing research questions/statements and selecting the appropriate methodology
- Attending to possible conflicts of interest (in your case it might be strong beliefs about certain provisions or models of healthcare in nursing and midwifery), as well as finan-cial obligation, personal relationships or affiliation with a third party (Taylor and Francis Group, 2012)
- Ensuring that you report all methodological issues honestly
- Respecting intellectual property as researchers have invested academic worth in the form of time and resources; therefore their work should be acknowledged
- Not fabricating or falsifying or misrepresenting data (Resnik, 2011)
- Endeavouring to avoid discrimination, particularly in selecting the criteria for evaluating the literature.

━━━━━━━━━━ **STUDENT ACTIVITY 5.2** ━━━━━━━━━━

In Chapter 2, there was an example of a student midwife called Jasmine. She was con-vinced her research was going to find that home is the place for women to give birth. This preconceived notion was based on Jasmine's observations in practice and from her own personal experience of having had a baby at home.

(Continued)

(Continued)

From this example, you can see that personal values and beliefs can pre-empt the findings of your research. Therefore, it is good practice to start by reflecting upon the clinical and/or personal experiences that are issues for concern. This will enable you to separate these clearly.

We would now like you to work with other students in your action learning set to:

- discuss the possible perceived biases you may have concerning your own individual research projects
- compare what you have declared as personal bias to what other students have seen as possible bias on your part as the researcher (refer to your reflective logs and research questions and/or statements that you have written)
- work out how you can minimize or avoid these biases (either on your own or with the help of other students).

From the above activity, you may find that declaring your own biases (based on your values and beliefs) is more difficult than you think because you need to be honest with yourself. Honesty requires you to avoid imposition of your own values and beliefs – in other words, your own ontological and epistemological position – on your research. It is only when you are honest with yourself that you can be truthful and fair with your data.

The main thrust of *truthfulness* is to avoid falsification or misrepresentation of data. Steneck (2002) states that your obligation as a researcher is not to deceive your colleagues and clients as they may use your findings for making decisions. *Fairness*, on the other hand, requires you to treat every research report that you read with respect and to honour intellectual property.

Another important consideration here is that researchers must provide fair inclusion of potential participants or groups and that participants or groups are not inappropriately excluded. Examples of this include attributes such as age, ethnicity, gender, culture and lack of capacity to consent. Similarly, in a comprehensive literature review you need to ensure that you have not excluded papers that you may consider inappropriate to your research on the basis of attributes such as philosophical stances, methodology or professional and disciplinary contexts.

5.2.2 The ethical principle of transparency

Figure 5.3 illustrates the three principles that define the concept of transparency. These are *accuracy*, *openness* and *accessibility*. In essence, transparency is to do with disclosure of all relevant stages of the research process. It is also about having a clear audit trail to show how accurate you have been in the conduct of the research project so that others can replicate the procedures.

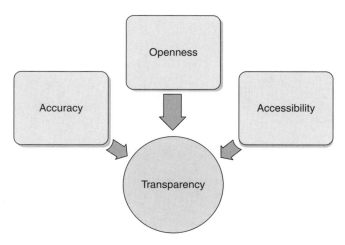

Figure 5.3 The key elements of transparency (adapted from Armstrong, 2005)

Of the three, *accuracy* perhaps is the core principle, as McHenry and Jureidini (2008) assert that health professionals and the public rely on the accuracy of published research. To ensure accuracy, there are some important factors you need to consider. These are:

- Researchers must establish transparency between their own philosophical position, the purpose of the research and the methodology
- The link between methodology and methods must be made explicit and transparent throughout the research process, especially in the development of evaluative criteria for critiquing, in analysis and interpretation of data, and in the dissemination of research findings.

In most research texts, *openness* refers mainly to two things: reporting on research in a responsible manner and acknowledging all those who have contributed to research. However, we need to add another point here, as openness also requires you to be open to criticism and to take steps to promote ethical practice in research (this is elaborated under accountability). *Accessibility*, on the other hand, requires that information is accurate and accessible when required. It is important that the researcher leaves an audit trail whereby the research process can be verified (Rolfe, 2006). This is further elaborated in Chapter 7.

5.2.3 The ethical principle of accountability

Accountability as an ethical dimension of the comprehensive literature review methodology is most important for two reasons: it recognizes the contribution

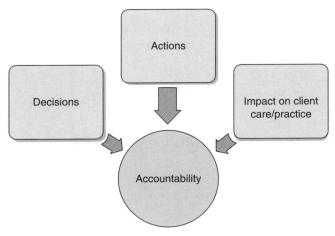

Figure 5.4   The key principles of accountability (adapted from Armstrong, 2005)

of research to evidence-based practice and it utilizes research evidence to inform policy and practice for the benefit of client care. Figure 5.4 shows the three key principles of accountability. These are *decisions*, *actions* and *impact on client care/ practice*.

Accountability lies not only with you as the researcher, but also with healthcare professionals. In the same vein that the Nursing and Midwifery Council (NMC) Code of Conduct (2008) speaks of the protection of the public, so, as a researcher, you need to take a conscious *decision* to foster public trust in the research evidence generated. Basically, this is about your performance as a researcher on the following three counts:

- The decisions that you will make on the evaluative criteria chosen for your analysis and the interpretation
- The decision to treat the data from someone else's literature with scholarly rigour (Davenport, 2010), i.e. your faithfulness in presenting these data as they feature in the text rather than in your own presuppositions (Sandelowski, 1986)
- The decision to report to the appropriate ethical committee if the papers you examined fall short of good ethical conduct in research. The notion of beneficence and malefi-cence is of significance here (as student researchers, you may choose to contact your research supervisor for advice on this matter).

The second and third key principles of accountability, *actions* and *impact on client care and practice* concern the utilization of your research to gain consent (as in the case of clients) or inform clinical decisions (as in the case of staff) or policy influencing practice. If your research aims to contribute to improving practice, then you need to ensure that your interpretation does not do a disservice to the clients and staff. You will also be looking to establish if the researchers of the papers examined are doing a disservice to clients. In some instances, you may set out to study an area that either lacks evidence or existing evidence may be outdated. Therefore, part of the action that you may take is disseminating your findings, as your comprehensive literature review may facilitate clinical decision making in areas where findings from empirical research or even systematic reviews are not appropriate.

The next section addresses the development of evaluative criteria for your literature review. In our experience, these criteria have enabled a more rigorous approach to assessing quality.

5.3 Defining Evaluative Criteria

A comprehensive literature review methodology handles both empirical and non-empirical literature. In other words, it adopts a pluralistic approach. It helps you, the researcher, to work with widely differing literature-based data. Therefore, the evaluative criteria need to be adaptable to the type of literature that you have selected.

There has been significant debate on the criteria for judging empirical research, particularly qualitative methodologies (Rolfe, 2006; Porter, 2007), but there is still very little beyond the generic research texts about the significance and application of ethics to comprehensive literature review methodology. It is important to note that, in the comprehensive literature review methodology, the usual ways in which criteria are applied to evaluate and establish quality may not be appropriate to evaluate published research and other forms of textual data.

In essence, critiquing the literature is about data analysis. In a comprehensive literature review methodology this involves stripping the research paper as a whole to its various components. It is important to note that critiquing is not a one-way system. It is an interrogative and dialogical process. Metaphorically speaking, you engage with the papers and allow the papers to engage with you. This is similar to the hermeneutic process (this will be further discussed in Chapter 6). To do this successfully and ethically, you need to have a clear set of criteria and to conduct your analysis in an ethical manner.

The critiquing stage of the literature involves making a judgement about whether it satisfies the principles defined above. Before doing so, you are required to define and set the evaluative criteria for making your judgement. This is a formal process and ought to be done systematically. A simple way of making your evaluative criteria explicit is via your data extraction tool, an example of which is given in Table 3.3 in Chapter 3. Student Activity 5.3 enables you to review some of the critique frameworks from which you can devise your own.

STUDENT ACTIVITY 5.3

A data extraction tool is simply a tool that will enable you to analyze your data in a systematic way. It should constitute sufficient criteria to enable you to assess the entire research process of the literature-based data. Our students in the past have indicated that it is a simple way of keeping data analysis manageable.

It is good practice to look at a few frameworks before you decide what evaluative criteria to include in your own data extraction tool. For examples of critique look at the following links:

Source of publication: journal

www.cybernurse.org.uk/research/Reading_and_Critiquing research.htm
http://library.ukc.ac.uk/library/info.subject/healthinfo/critapprais.htm
www.york.ac.uk/inst/crd/pdf/Systematic.Review.pdf
www.nursingplanet.com/...Research/critiquing_nursing_health

Source of publication: website

www.uwindsor.ca.units/leddy/leddy.nsf/Evaluatingwebsite
www.library.council.edu/dinuris/ref/research/webeval.htm

Look at two or three of the above examples of frameworks and consider the similarities and differences. Make a judgement on their strengths and limitations. Share your findings with other students.

You may find that the choice of evaluative criteria to include in your data extraction tools is very much a personal preference. It is what you are familiar with and what will enable you to conduct a fair judgement that counts.

The set of evaluative criteria detailed in the following sections are only guidelines and should be used with a degree of flexibility. The aim is to allow you to judge each piece of literature on its own merit.

5.3.1 Source of publication

In most critique frameworks, the source of publication features as the first criterion. At first glance, this criterion appears to request details such as name of the journal, its peer-reviewed status and impact factor (the frequency with which the journal article has been cited). These add to the credibility of the journal and the trust placed in the research evidence published therein. Other factors that you need to investigate include:

1 **Publication guidelines** – This is to determine if the journals provide adequate guidelines for the researchers. It will enable you to assess whether the researcher has been restricted to publish only certain aspects of the research due to word limits. This may then be a good reason for you to contact the author for further information.

2 **Multiple authorship** – In the case of multiple authorship, there should be clear details about each author's responsibilities (Resnik and Master, 2011). Although in your work you will be the single author, we are increasingly seeing papers with multiple authorship. You need to be mindful of issues such as the contribution each author has made and who has ownership of the ideas (Clyde, 2005). If there are funding agencies involved, there may be a duty to promote their product, which might or might not be in the interest of client care. This is an issue of accountability.

Student Example 5.1   Publication guidelines for the International Journal of Obstetrics and Gynaecology

Look at the publication guidelines for the above journal at: www.bjog.org/view/0/authorInformation.html. Take note of the restrictions placed on authors by publishers. Note where the publisher's requirement for each author's specific contributions to the study is stated (Resnik and Master, 2011).

5.3.2 Title of the paper

The title is an important feature of any research paper. Often the research question is used as the title of research paper. Here you will need to examine if the title conveys what the study seeks to address. This might be difficult to uncover at the initial stage of your evaluation, therefore you may need to return to this criterion after you have read the entire paper in order to make a fair and accurate judgement.

5.3.3 The author/researcher

This criterion is often poorly examined or overlooked. Most critiques that address this criterion have tended to limit the evaluation to credentials such as the qualifications of the researchers. Undoubtedly this is important, but there are major aspects pertaining to the authorship that you need to consider, as follows:

1 **Disciplinary and professional contexts of the author/researcher** – As you have learnt in Chapter 2, we bring with us our different perspectives to our area of practice. This may stem from our professional and/or disciplinary contexts, such as medicine or anthropology. It is therefore important that such biographical details are made clear.

2 **The contribution of each author/researcher** – In the case of multiple authors, it is necessary to assess each author's contribution to the study, such as contribution to the design of the study, data collection or analysis, or writing the final report. In most quantitative studies it is normal practice to engage a statistician to analyze data.

5.3.4 The researchers' philosophical basis

As you have seen in Chapter 2, the philosophical basis of research refers to two distinct aspects: ontology and epistemology. This is influenced by the three contexts identified in Figure 2.2, namely historical or philosophical context, disciplinary or professional context and social or everyday life context. Part of stripping away the data includes seeking out the researchers' ontological and epistemological position. You can do so in two ways:

1   Establishing the researchers' closeness to the subject of the study (Meyrick, 2006). For example, have they allowed their beliefs, values and experience to shape their choice of methodology and methods? This will ultimately influence their findings.
2   Declaring the researchers' philosophical positions. This is good practice in situating the research, formulating the research question/statement and identifying the chosen methodology, as mentioned in Chapter 2. Do not be surprised if this is not stated as it is an aspect that is neglected in most publications.

5.3.5 Research question/statement

The research question/statement serves an important role in any research studies in so far as it will determine the entire course of the research. Here you will examine whether the research question/statement and the process through which this is formulated are made explicit. There should be congruence between the research question/statement and the selection of methodology and methods. In other words, can you identify how the research question has led to the methodology and methods? If so, how do they fit together?

5.3.6 Aim of the study

This criterion is not always expressed clearly as it may also be called: 'Terms of reference', 'Statement of purpose' or 'Intention of the study'. It does not matter which expression is used, the important point here is that the aim of the study needs to be congruent with the title, methodology and methods. Examples of questions for you to ask are:

1   Is the aim of the study stated and, if so, in what form?
2   How does the aim, statement of purpose or intention of the study relate to the title, research question, methodology and methods?

5.3.7 Literature review

According to Boote and Beile (2005), researchers must have a good understanding of the literature and previous research conducted in their proposed area of study. As part of the process, it is customary for a preliminary literature review to be conducted for the following reasons:

1 To see what research has been done on the subject and what claims the researchers have made.
2 To see if there are any gaps existing in the knowledge of the subject.
3 To see what methodology the researchers have used and its appropriateness for that study.
4 To see if existing research confirms or supports the research question.

It is also important to look at the currency and source of the literature. Sometimes dated literature may be necessary when a historical context is relevant for the subject, or where there is an absence of recent research on the subject of study.

Student Example 5.2 Congruence between the research question/statement and the selection of methodology and methods

Read the abstract below from the following research paper:

Gorter, K.J., Tuytel, G.J. and de Leeuw, R.R. (2011) Opinions of patients with type 2 diabetes about responsibility, setting targets and willingness to take medication: a cross-sectional survey, *Patient Education and Counselling*, 84(1), 56–61.

Objective

To assess opinions and their determinants of patients with type 2 diabetes about responsibility for managing their diabetes, setting treatment targets and willingness taking medication.

Methods

Questionnaire survey carried out in general practices and outpatient clinics across the Netherlands.

Outcomes

Opinions about responsibility, targets and medication. Multinomial logistic regression analysis.

Results

Data of 994 consecutive persons were analyzed (mean age 65 years; 54% males). Of these, 62% agreed to take responsibility for their diabetes. In

(Continued)

(Continued)

the opinion of 89%, the setting of targets should be by or in cooperation with their physician or nurse and 40% were willing to take tablets until all targets were attained. Patients who perceived dysfunction by barriers to activity did not agree to take responsibility (Odds Ratio 3.68; 1.65–8.19). Patients with complications preferred to set targets in cooperation with their physician or nurse (Odds Ratio 1.98; 1.03–3.80). Males were more willing to take tablets until all targets were attained (Odds Ratio 1.62; 1.17–2.25).

Conclusion

Not all patients want to take responsibility for their diabetes or taking all necessary tablets, especially those with barriers to activity or complications.

Practice implications

Doctors and nurses should ask for patients' opinions about responsibility and treatment goals before starting education.

This research is of a *survey* design using *questionnaires* as the method of data collection. This was clearly stated under the heading of methods. The *title* of the article gives you the additional information of the type of survey conducted – *cross-sectional* (i.e. the survey was taken at the same point in time).

The research is also in line with a *quantitative* paradigm as *outcome measures* (responsibility, targets and medication) are indicated as well as the use of *statistics* (multinominal logistic regression analysis). These variables are also picked up in the reporting of the results.

The final and important issue to note is how the researchers have stated the *objectives* of their research. Their research statement reflects the 'quantitativeness' of the research as the '*opinions and determinants of patients*' are quantifiable variables. This is congruent with the rest of the research design and reporting.

5.3.8 Methodology

Often the terms 'methodology' and 'methods' are used synonymously. It is important to distinguish between methodology and methods. We would like to remind you of the definitions of these terms, as stated in Chapter 1.

Methodology is the strategy, plan of action, process or design lying behind the choice and use of particular methods and linking the choice and use of methods to the desired outcomes.

Methods are the techniques and procedures used to gather and analyse data related to some research question or hypothesis. (Crotty, 2003: 3)

In other words, methodology is the relationship between philosophy and the approach to research design. It is important that you elicit whether the methodology employed has been stated; and if a philosophical position is stated, you need to examine if it fits with the methodology.

Student Example 5.3   **Relationship between philosophical position of the researcher and the methodology and methods of the research**

Read the abstract below from the following research paper:

Fleming, S.E. and Vandermause, R. (2011) Grand multiparae's evolving experiences of birthing and technology in US hospitals, *Journal of Obstetric, Gynecologic and Neonatal Nursing*, 40(6), 742–752.

Objective

To explore the nature of birthing in United States (US) hospitals from 1973–2007 and to explicate and interpret common, often overlooked, birthing experiences and nursing (*midwifery*) care.

Design

A Heideggerian phenomenological approach utilizing in-depth interviews.

Setting

Participants' homes in Washington, Idaho, and Oregon.

Participants

A purposive sample of grand multiparaes ($N = 14$).

Methods

Data were collected via open conversational interviews of 60–90 minutes recorded on digital media and completion of a demographic and birth attribute form. Field notes and interpretive commentary were used as additional data sources and were analyzed using an established Heideggerian approach.

Results

The participants came from diverse religious and ethnic backgrounds and experienced 116 births (8.29 births per woman, 79% unmedicated), a

(Continued)

(Continued)

Cesarean rate of 6%, and a breastfeeding rate of 99% with a mean duration of 12 months. Two overarching patterns emerged: pursuing the 'good birth': a safe passage for baby and being in-and-out of control: body, technology, others. Each pattern subsumed several overlapping themes. The first pattern revealed that women often desire a good birth in the safety of a hospital by navigating their options prior to and during the birth. The second pattern revealed a common, yet often unachievable, desire by all of those involved in the process to control birth.

Conclusion

Harmonizing an exchange of ideas in a technologically advanced environment prevalent in hospitals today can increase the quality of intrapartum care. Encouraging anchored companions and promoting normal physiological birth will make hospitals places where women can experience a good birth and feel safe.

As you learned in Chapter 2, the philosophical position of the researcher needs to be congruent with the methodology and methods. This may not always be evident in the research paper. In this paper it is not stated. Although this is a weakness, it does not mean that the research is flawed. The next thing to look at is the relationship between the purpose of the research and the methodology.

The research is a phenomenological study which uses a Heideggerian approach. The method of data collection and sampling are in keeping with the philosophical basis of phenomenology. The term 'field notes', mentioned under methods, is a characteristic of ethnography, so this can be misleading. The point to remember is that methods of data collection in qualitative research cross-cut methodological approaches. In that respect the research is in line with phenomenology.

The results are presented in a combined way, using basic statistics and thematic representation. By inference, the researcher has used a deductive and inductive approach to arriving at the results presented. Qualitative research does not employ the principles of statistics, so the importance here is that the researcher has blended elements of both qualitative and quantitative approaches to present the findings.

Summarizing the last two sections, the overarching criterion is to establish the presence of congruence when you are evaluating a research paper. There are certain characteristics that you should look for to establish if the methodology is commensurate with the research question/statement. This will vary depending on the types of literature that your comprehensive literature review scrutinizes. If a piece of research has used a quantitative approach, such as a survey or a randomized controlled trial, you will be looking for a research statement or a set of hypotheses along with a different set of characteristics in that research. Similarly, a qualitative approach, such as a phenomenological or an ethnographic design, will have a research question or set of questions, along with different characteristics that is in line with a qualitative paradigm.

5.3.9 The sample

The sample is another important dimension of the research process. The type and characteristics of the sample are dependent upon the type of research. For example, quantitative research uses large samples, whereas with qualitative research the sample is generally small. The sample will affect the quality of data collected and in turn will influence the quality of the research findings.

The important point to look out for is consistency in the type of sampling used in the selection process: for example, the use of randomization in quantitative research and the use of purposive sampling in qualitative research. You also need to examine whether the sample and the method of selecting that sample are commensurate with the study: in other words, whether they link to the research question/statement. Other questions to consider are:

- Is the size of the sample appropriate?
- Is the size of the sample a fair representation of the population?
- Have the authors described their sampling strategy and provided the rationale and the theories to support their selection?

5.3.10 Data collection

The question that you need to ask here is not only how data were collected but also whether the data are consistent with the research question/statement, methodology and sample. In addition to ensuring consistency between all the factors mentioned, you should examine whether the researcher has made the method of data collection explicit: for example, the use of a single method of data collection or a combination of methods.

A quantitative approach may use self-designed or pre-designed tests, scales or scoring tools. There may be questionnaires only or a combination of structured interviews and/or structured observations. At the same time, it is just as important to match the research design to the choice of data collection method(s). If the study is a survey, then a questionnaire is the most common and appropriate method of collecting data.

Assessing method of data collection in qualitative studies may not be so straightforward. As you have learned in Chapter 1, there are a number of research approaches to qualitative studies. Examples of these are phenomenology, ethnography, grounded theory, narrative inquiry, and so forth. Each of these has specific methods of data collection. In phenomenological studies, the essence of which is to explore the lived experience of the research participants, the usual method of data collection is open-ended interviews, which may be repeated with the same participants on more than one occasion.

A final point to make is that data collection and analysis are frequently concomitant in qualitative research. This means that the researcher in the course of a study may make changes in the technique or focus of data collection and may undertake some analysis before data collection is complete. In such cases, researchers should provide a detailed justification for doing so. As the reviewer, you should then be able to judge if the changes made during data collection were warranted.

Student Example 5.4 The appropriateness of sample size, sampling type and methods of data collection

Read the abstract below which is taken from the following research paper (extracted online) ncbi.nlm.gov/pubmed/22211526

Machin, A.I., Machin, T. and Pearson, P. (2012) 'Maintaining equilibrium in professional role identity: a grounded theory study of health visitors' perceptions of their changing professional practice context', *Journal of Advanced Nursing*.

Aims

> This article reports the study of a group of United Kingdom health visitors' interactions with their changing practice context, focusing on role identity and influences on its stability.

Background

> United Kingdom policies have urged health visitors to refocus their role as key public health nurses. Reduced role identity clarity precipitated the emergence of different models of health visiting public health work. An inconsistent role standard can lead to role identity fragmentation and conflict across a group. It may precipitate individual role crisis, affecting optimum role performance.

Methods

> Seventeen health visitors in two United Kingdom community healthcare organizations participated in a grounded theory study, incorporating constant comparative analysis. Direct observations and individual interviews were undertaken between 2002 and 2008.

Results/findings

Four interlinked categories emerged: professional role identity (core category); professional role in action; inter-professional working; and local micro-systems for practice; each influencing participants' sense of identity and self-worth. The Role Identity Equilibrium Process explains interactive processes occurring at different levels of participants' practice.

Conclusion

Re-establishing equilibrium and consistency in health visiting identity is a priority. This study's findings have significance for other nurses and health professionals working in complex systems, affected by role change and challenges to role identity.

This qualitative study has used a *grounded theory* research design, which is made explicit in the *title* of the article and under the heading of *methods* in the abstract of this paper. It is also evident from the title and methods section of the abstract that the target population is health visitors. Although the *sampling type* was not declared, it can be assumed that the 17 health visitors from the two UK community healthcare organizations were *purposely selected*. It is not untypical that a *small sample* of 17 was chosen for data collection since *both direct observations and individual interviews were conducted over a six-year period*. Despite the small sample, this would have generated a large amount of data, as is expected from a qualitative study.

Equally importantly, you should elicit how data was recorded, such as the use of scoring tools, self-recorded diaries, audiotapes or videotapes. There are two points to consider here:

1 **The use of more than one researcher for data collection** – The issue of inter-rater reliability is a key consideration with quantitative research (in particular). You will need to identify in the research literature itself whether this has been declared and dealt with.
2 **The use of a transcriber** – It is normal practice to have a transcriber. Transcription is more often than not carried out by a person other than the researcher, usually a secretary. There are limitations here, in so far as the quality of the transcript will depend on the instructions given by the researcher. Other important factors to consider relate to participants' behaviour, such as facial expressions, intonations, laughter, that describe aspects of lived expressions that cannot be captured in transcripts (Barnacle, 2005). The problem here is that when such important factors are lost, the quality of data may be jeopardized, leading to misinterpretation of findings.

5.3.11 Data analysis

In any research paper, the data analysis section begins by describing the methods used for analysis.

In quantitative research, the researcher should describe the statistical tests used and the statistical analysis undertaken. There are a great variety of statistical tests in the form of software packages that are available to the quantitative researcher. There are two types of statistics: descriptive and inferential statistics. Descriptive statistics describe the results of the study and summarize them in a clear manner (usual in diagrammatic format). Inferential statistics serve two main purposes: to see whether relationships between variables exist and to establish the precise nature of the relationship (Parahoo, 2006). The strength of inferential statistics is to allow findings from one research sample to be generalized to the whole population. As the reviewer of these pieces of quantitative research you need to be mindful of how researchers can lie with statistics. If at any time you are unsure about the statistical techniques employed in a piece of research, you can either contact the author or consult your own statistician on the matter.

In qualitative research there are also a wide variety of methods used for analysis, such as content, thematic or discourse analysis. The essence of qualitative data analysis is to interpret the data from both the subject's and the researcher's points of view. The strength of the findings generated is unique to that situation, time and person(s). The qualitative researcher needs to be explicit about the steps of interpretation. It is important for the researcher to constantly assess the relationship between the research study, the methodology and the researcher's own philosophical stance.

The final task for you here is to assess that the method of data analysis employed by the researcher is consistent, not only with the methodology and methods, but also with the research question/statements and the aims and objectives of that research.

5.3.12 The findings

It is crucial to include sufficient detail about how findings are arrived at and presented. The presentation of findings will depend upon the type of research approach (quantitative, qualitative or mixed methodology). The task here is to assess how the findings or results section is structured. No matter what methodology the researcher is using, the findings need to be described in a systematic way.

In quantitative research, the findings or results are presented in tables or other diagrammatic representation. It is essential that these findings are accompanied by explanatory texts. The best way of presenting the findings is in terms of the research statement or aims and objectives of the research.

In qualitative research, the findings are presented in words (per verbatim). Its purpose is to provide 'rich description' of what the participants have relayed to the researcher in the form of data, and the findings must be grounded in the participants' subjective meaning. This will reflect the voice of the participants and the extent to which the research makes a contribution to new knowledge and our understanding of that knowledge. The task here is to examine whether there are sufficient quotes from the data – i.e. the findings need to include per verbatim what the participants have stated. It is also normal practice to present the findings of qualitative research in the form of the researcher's own interpretation.

In mixed methodology papers there needs to be a balanced approach that reflects considerable attention to both approaches of research.

STUDENT ACTIVITY 5.4

This exercise allows you to focus on the method of data analysis and the processes used in this stage of the research. It also asks questions of you when you are assessing the research findings.

Choose a quantitative research paper, a qualitative research paper and one using a mixed methodology. Go through the following questions systematically:

For quantitative research

• Are the methods of analysis stated and consistent with the aim of the study and the methodology?
• How are the results presented?
• Are they in tables or other diagrammatic representations?
• Are there explanatory texts that accompany these diagrammatic representations?
• Are the findings or results presented in terms of the identified research statement or corresponding aims and objectives?

For qualitative research

• Are the methods of analysis stated and consistent with the aims of the study and the methodology?
• Are there sufficient quotes from the data generated by the participants?
• Are you able to trace which quotes are generated from which participants?
• Have the researcher's presented their findings in themes?
• How have they arrived at the reported themes?
• Is the process described (or illustrated) clearly?
• Is the researcher's reflexivity evident?

For mixed methodology

• Is the appropriate method of data analysis employed in both methodological approaches?
• Is there a balance between both methodological approaches?
  (Plus all the questions above)

5.3.13 Discussion and conclusion

This is the final part of the research report as the researchers bring the study together. It is in this section that the researcher discusses the findings in the light of what is already known. In other words, the researcher should interrogate the findings with what they have discussed in the preliminary literature review. The researcher should also return to the research questions/statements and relate these to the discussion of the study. The purpose is to ensure that the research questions/statements have been adequately addressed.

In every good conclusion, the researcher should indicate how the findings impact upon practice and suggest recommendations that may enhance or be used to develop practice. More often than not, a researcher ends with further questions for future research related to the studied topic.

5.4 How to evaluate non-empirical literature (grey literature)

You may have chosen the following non-empirical literature:

- Policy documents
- Audit documents
- Theory (theories). For example, a theory that explains a physiological process that has led to our understanding of how the human body functions and thus provides a basis for care, such as the physiology of gastric emptying and the impact on peri-operative care.

In addition to what has already been explored in the previous sections on evaluating empirical literature, there is specific information that you will need to address when examining grey literature. Policies are formed and implemented to improve client care. In the evaluation of policies you will need to be looking at the development of the policy. The process involved in policy development is similar to that involved in empirical studies. It starts with the identification of a problem that leads to actions taken by policy makers. In a local context, this will include the Trust or, in a national context, the government. Therefore, the principles used to evaluate government policies can also be applied to local audits. For both policies and audits, the motive behind their development needs to be understood.

Critique of theories, however, presents a different challenge and most of the time theories underpinning our understanding of, for instance, physiology and physiological processes are taken for granted. Theories that can be applied to practice, such as those in nursing and midwifery, will be judged by their applicability and how they withstand the test of time.

The following sets of questions provide some guidelines upon which the evaluative criteria can be based:

Critique of policy documents

- Who were involved in the decision-making process (e.g. think tanks, interest groups and committees)?
- What are the factors that led to the policy development?
- Are those factors representative of the general population's view?
- What is the evidence and source of evidence that underpins the policy?
- What is the impact upon practice in relation to the implementation of the policy?
- What are the limitations (i.e. the resource issues both in terms of manpower and finance)?

Critique of audit

- What are the factors that led to the necessity of the audit?
- Who was involved in the audit?
- What is the evidence or source of evidence that underpins the audit?
- Is there an identified framework?
- Are the standards set appropriate?
- Is there consistency between the standards and the purpose of the audit?
- Do the findings of the audit impact upon practice and client care?
- Can the findings inform future research?

Critique of theories

- How up to date are the theories?
- Upon what evidence do the authors base their authority?
- Is the source of evidence research-based, anecdotal or clinical expertise?
- (If it is research) Was it conducted using human participants?
- (If the research was used on participants other than humans) Can the theories constructed be applied to human conditions?

================ **STUDENT ACTIVITY 5.5** ================

Choose from *one* of the following pieces of grey literature:

1 Government policy

Midwifery 2020 Programme: Core Role of the Midwife Workstream Final Report (31 March 2010), available at: www.midwifery2020.org/documents/2020/Core_Role.pdf

(Continued)

(Continued)

2 Local audit

Medicine Use Review Audit, NHS Leeds 2009–2010 (April 2010), available at: www.leeds.
nhs.uk/About-us/Information%20for%20Professionals/Medicines%20Management/
mur-audit.htm

3 Theory

Mendelson's Theory on Gastric Aspiration (1946): a PatientPlus article (December 2010),
available at: www.patient.co.uk/doctor/Mendelson's-Syndrome.htm

Scrutinize the chosen publication and answer the questions set out in the appropriate list
on evaluating grey literature (see page 109). Compare your findings with another student
and share these with other students in your action learning set who looked at different
types of grey literature.

In order to do an in-depth and ethically based critique you need to read and
re-read your data before you can identify themes. In the next chapter we take
you a stage further and define the process of themes identification.

End-of-Chapter Learning Points

We hope that you have found this chapter helpful in understanding the tenets of ethics in literature-based research methodology. It will also help you to
conduct your own comprehensive literature review in an ethical manner. The
following are some of the key points highlighted in this chapter:

1 Ethics are an important aspect of a comprehensive literature review methodology and in conducting your review you need to keep in mind the principles
   of ethics to ensure good practice in research.
2 Ethical considerations are important and are based on integrity, transparency
   and accountability in order to show rigour in your research project. These
   concepts enable us to consider our obligations when we utilize literature-
   based data as raw data.
3 A comprehensive literature review methodology handles a diversity of literature-based data and it is important that a flexible approach to analysis is
   considered.
4 An important challenge in conducting a comprehensive literature review
   methodology is to recognize the relevance of rigour and your responsibility

to consider ethical issues beyond its applicability to empirical research. Failure to do so may lead to charges of misconduct in research.

5 There are definite evaluative criteria for both empirical and non-empirical literature. They should be considered in the depth described in this chapter in order to arrive at a fair and trustworthy analysis. You should exercise flexibility in adapting these criteria to your own research.

References

On research governance and methodological rigour

Armstrong, E. (2005) *Integrity, Transparency and Accountability in Public Administration: Recent Trends, Regional and International Developments and Emerging Issues.* http:www.upan1.un.org/intradoc/groups/public/.../un/upan020955.pdf.

Boote, D.N. and Beile, P.(2005) 'Scholars before researchers: on the centrality of the dissertation literature review in research preparation', *Educational Researchers*, 34(6), 3–15.

Crotty, M. (2003) *The Foundations of Social Research: Meaning and Perspective in Social Research.* London: Sage.

Davenport, P. (2010) *Report of the Expert Panel on Research Integrity.* Ottawa: Council of Canadian Academies. Available at: www.scienceadvice.ca.

Department of Health (2001) *Research Governance Framework for England.* London: Department of Health.

Meyrick, J. (2006) 'What is good qualitative research? A first step towards a comprehensive approach to judging rigour/quality', *Journal of Health Psychology*, 11(5), 799–808.

Porter, S. (2007) 'Validity, trustworthiness and rigour: reasserting realism in qualitative research', *Journal of Advancing Nursing*, 60(1), 79–86.

Rolfe, G. (2006) 'Validity, trustworthiness and rigour: quality and the idea of qualitative research', *Journal of Advanced Nursing*, 53, 304–310.

Sandelowski, M. (1986) 'The problem of rigor in qualitative research', *Advance Nursing Science*, 8, 27–37.

On ethics and policy

Beauchamp, T.L. and Childress, J.F. (2008) *Principles of Biomedical Ethics* (6th edn). New York: Oxford University Press.

McHenry, L.B. and Jureidini, J.N. (2008) 'Industry-sponsored ghostwriting in clinical trial reporting: a case study', *Accountability in Research*, 15, 152–167.

Nursing and Midwifery Council (2008) *The Code: Standards of Conduct, Performance and Ethics for Nurses and Midwives.* London: NMC.

Resnik, D.B. (2011) *What is Ethics in Research and Why is it Important?* Available at: www.niehs.nih.gov/research/resources/bioethics/whatis.cfm (accessed 23 January 2012).

Resnik, D.B. and Master, Z. (2011) 'Authorship policies of bioethics journals', *Journal of Medical Ethics*, 37, 424–428.

Steneck, N.H. (2002) 'Assessing the integrity of publicly supported research', in N.H. Steneck, and M.D. Scheetz (eds), *Investigating Research Integrity: Preceedings of the*

First ORI Research Conference on Research Integrity. Washington, DC: Office of Research Integrity.

Taylor and Francis Group (2012) *Accountability in Research – Policies and Quality Assurance.* Available at: www.tandf.co.uk/journals/authors/gacraiuth.asp

Economic & Social Research Council (2011) *The Research Ethics Guidebook: A Resource for Social Scientist.* Swindson: ESRC. www.ethicsguidebook.ac.uk/Literature-reviews-and-systematuc-reviews-99

On research and evidence-based practice

Barnacle, R. (2005) 'Interpreting interpretation: a phenomenological perspective on phenenography', in J.A. Bowden and P. Green (eds), *Doing Developmental Phenomenography.* Melbourne: RMIT University Press.

Clyde, A.L. (2005) '*The basis for evidence-based practice: evaluating the research evidence*', *New Library World*, 107(5/6), 180–192. Available at: www.ifla.org/IVfla71/Programee.thm.

Fleming, S.E. and Vandermause, R. (2011) 'Grand multiparae's evolving experiences of birthing and technology in US hospitals', *Journal of Obstetric, Gynecologic and Neonatal Nursing*, 40(6), 742–752.

Gorter, K.J., Tuytel, G.J. and de Leeuw, R.R. (2011) 'Opinions of patients with type 2 diabetes about responsibility, setting targets and willingness to take medication: a cross-sectional survey', *Patient Education and Counselling*, 84(1), 56–61.

Machin, A.I., Machin, T. and Pearson, P. (2012) 'Maintaining equilibrium in professional role identity: a grounded theory study of health visitors' perceptions of their changing professional practice context', *Journal of Advanced Nursing*, 68(7), 1526–37. ncbi.nlm. gov/pubmed/22211526

Parahoo, K. (2006) *Nursing Research: Principles, Process and Issues* (2nd edn). Basingstoke: Palgrave Macmillan.

Websites

Critique Frameworks

www.cybernurse.org.uk/research/Reading_and_Critiquing research.htm
http://library.ukc.ac.uk/library/info.subject/healthinfo/critapprais.htm
www.york.ac.uk/inst/crd/pdf/Systematic.Review.pdf
www.nursingplanet.com/...Research/critiquing_nursing_health
www.uwindsor.ca.units/leddy/leddy.nsf/Evaluatingwebsite
www.library.council.edu/dinuris/ref/research/webeval.htm
International Journal of Obstetrics and Gynaecology – www.bjog.org/view/0/authorInformation. html

Medicine Use Review Audit, NHS Leeds 2009–2010 (April 2010). Available at: www.leeds. nhs.uk/About-us/Information%20for%20Professionals/Medicines%20Management/ mur-audit.htm (accessed 5 February 2012).

Mendelson's Theory on Gastric Aspiration (1946): a PatientPlus article (December 2010). Available at: www.patient.co.uk/doctor/Mendelson's-Syndrome.htm (accessed 5 February 2012).

Midwifery 2020 Programme: Core Role of the Midwife Workstream Final Report (31 March 2010). Available at: www.midwifery2020.org/documents/2020/Core_Role.pdf (accessed 5 February 2012).

SIX
Analysis and Synthesis of Literature-Based Data

┌─ **Aim and objectives** ─┐

The aim of this chapter is to explore the processes of analysis and synthesis in the comprehensive literature review methodology. By the end of this chapter you will be able to:

- Identify the processes involved in the analysis of literature-based data
- Understand the meaning of theme
- Know the techniques involved in identifying and developing themes by engaging with the data in an iterative process
- Synthesize themes from analyzed data and show how you make the transition from one stage of analysis to synthesis
- Demonstrate critical reasoning.

6.1 Introduction

In this chapter we explore the processes of data analysis and synthesis in comprehensive literature review methodology. These are an important and complex part of the interpretive process in research. They involve the identification of themes and their synthesis, upon which new insights will be achieved. All researchers thus have a responsibility to ensure that this is carried out in a robust, trustworthy and competent manner. The three principles of ethics – integrity, transparency and accountability – introduced in Chapter 5, will enable you to ensure your analysis and synthesis is worthy of trust. Because the comprehensive literature review incorporates data from a plurality of methodology and source, the approach to analysis and synthesis needs to draw on both positivist and interpretivist episte-mology. Here, we are not suggesting that you undertake a combination of meta-analysis and meta-synthesis, but you need some form of simple quantification, particularly when assigning degrees of importance to categories, and preliminary stages of interpretation when developing themes.

It is therefore crucial to follow a systematic approach to the processes of analysis and synthesis, which we will explore in the following stages:

1 Defining the theoretical underpinning of comprehensive literature review data analysis and synthesis.
2 Defining the term 'theme' to contextualize the analysis and synthesis of comprehensive literature review data.
3 The process of developing and synthesizing themes.

These stages are vitally important and should not be underestimated. You need to set aside a realistic period of time to do it well. Your supervisor will be able to provide the necessary guidance on developing a realistic timetable or Gantt chart (see Chapter 8).

6.2 Defining the theoretical underpinning of comprehensive literature review data analysis and synthesis

In the analysis and synthesis of literature-based data the researcher starts by ask-ing the simple question: what do these collections of studies have to say? Before launching into an answer, you need to re-examine your philosophical stand-point by focusing on the research question(s) or statement(s) that you have writ-ten at the start of your research. This will help to set the scene for the processes of analysis and synthesis.

The pluralistic stance is the backbone of the comprehensive literature review methodology. It is our intention to bring together an eclectic approach to the analysis and synthesis stages. As stated in Chapter 3, there are a number of established theoretical approaches to analyze and synthesize literature-based data. Meta-analyses, employed by systematic reviewers, aim to bring together results of large numbers of quantitative studies. Meta-ethnography, meta-study, meta-theory and mixed research synthesis are examples of approaches to synthesize findings of qualitative studies (Paterson et al., 2001; Whittemore and Knafl, 2005; Popay, 2006; Sandelowski et al., 2007). In this chapter we draw on the influences of two theoretical approaches, *constant comparative method* and *hermeneutical exegesis*, to underpin the analysis and synthesis of literature-based data. We believe that both approaches bring openness to the interpretive processes. The following sections will focus on contextualizing the processes of data analysis and synthesis in the comprehensive literature review methodology by:

- defining the terms analysis and synthesis so as to provide a clear differentiation of these two processes
- providing a brief overview of the constant comparative method as an approach to analysis
- providing a brief overview of hermeneutical exegesis as an approach to synthesis.

6.2.1 Defining analysis and synthesis

When embarking upon the analysis and synthesis of your data, it is important to be clear what these two processes involve as there are distinct steps in each. From our experiences, analysis is the 'art and science' of examining the key features of the literature. This process entails inquiring into each key feature separately in order to gain a better understanding of how they fit together. As you will already know, the key features of each piece of literature include: title, author/researcher(s), philosophical basis, research question, literature review, methodology, sample, data collection, data analysis, findings, discussion and conclusion. You will have already entered this information in your data extraction sheet. The framework for analysis proposed in this book is the constant comparative method, which will be further elaborated in this chapter.

Synthesis, on the other hand, is 'the process or the result of building up separate elements, especially ideas into a connected whole which leads to theory building' (Oxford Dictionaries, 1990: 1238). We endorse this definition as the 'art and science' of putting back together the information that you have obtained from the analysis of your data into a wider interpretive framework. The framework for synthesis proposed in this book is hermeneutical exegesis, which will be further elaborated in this chapter.

6.2.2 Constant comparative method: the analytical approach

Constant comparative method in the process of analysis is the main characteristic of grounded theory. In this approach, as the term implies, theory is grounded in the data. In other words, it is generated from the data and develops during the actual research (Strauss and Corbin, 1994). According to Glaser and Strauss (1967), a key feature of grounded theory is the movement from substantive theories, grounded in a particular research context, to a more generic formal theory which can be applied in a broader context. It differs from other research approaches in that its inductively derived theory is based directly on the data rather than hypothesis testing (Glaser, 1978; Strauss and Corbin, 1994). Charmaz (2006) points out that the main thrust of grounded theory is to discover theory that is grounded in the research participants' personalized narrative of their experiences. Therefore, in the case of literature review methodology, theory is grounded in the literature-based data. The process of constant comparison is necessary to uncover the meaning that the findings of the literature hold. Its application to comprehensive literature review methodology is illustrated in Figure 6.1.

To summarize, in the constant comparative method, comparison is made between or among groups of people (literature-based data) within the subject of inquiry (Morse and Field, 1995). The constant comparative method in effect allows the researcher to identify patterns and the relationship between these patterns (Glaser, 1992). It involves *going back and forth* between the data or findings from the literature. This is what is also referred to as the iterative process. In comprehensive literature review methodology you will be engaging with the literature-based data in a similar fashion. Student Example 6.1 illustrates our point.

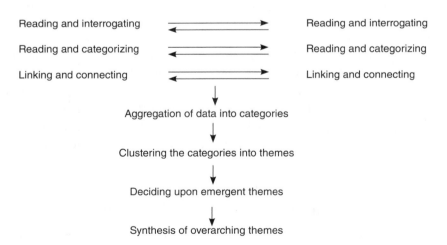

Figure 6.1 The iterative process of constant comparative analysis (adapted from Miles and Huberman, 1994)

Student Example 6.1 The use of the iterative process in identifying categories

In this example, we are using research on the prevention and detection of bowel cancer to illustrate the iterative process. We have highlighted some key findings from five pieces of research on bowel cancer:

Paper 1: Center et al. (2009) – worldwide trend analysis

The screening of bowel cancer has shown that early detection decreases mortality rates in developed countries by as much as 30% and the benefits of national and international bowel cancer screening programmes are irrefutable.

Paper 2: Goodyear et al. (2008) – retrospective trend analysis

Increased public awareness through the UK bowel cancer screening project in the West Midlands has positive impacts, such as attenuated emergency admissions, treatment and reduced mortality rates from bowel cancer.

Paper 3: Chapple et al. (2008) – qualitative interviews of the public

The uptake of the UK bowel cancer screening project in the form of faecal occult blood testing has been disappointing in some areas. More information on screening methods and people's experiences may increase participation by the public.

Paper 4: von Wagner et al. (2009) – national trend analysis

The average uptake of the UK bowel cancer screening project in the form of faecal occult blood testing has been low.

Paper 5: Simon et al. (2011) – qualitative interviews of healthcare professionals

Healthcare professionals believe that information about cancer should focus on improvements achieved through preventing and treating cancer.

The first step is to return to your research question(s) or statement(s). In this example, the research statement and question are:

- *There are differences between the public and healthcare professionals in their viewpoints on the prevention and detection of bowel cancer.*
- *How do the public and professionals feel about the way bowel cancer is prevented and detected?*

(Continued)

With the above in mind, you then proceed to go back and forth between the data or findings from the literature to see if you can identify categories. This can be in the form of similar and/or conflicting characteristics.

By grouping these together, you can see if there are areas of data that are missing. This may require you to return to the data searching stage. In the above example, research on the public's and healthcare professionals' viewpoints on bowel cancer screening is lacking. You may therefore need to return to your data extraction/summary table to see if there are data that you have not picked up or perhaps might not appear to be relevant initially. You may also need to widen your search criteria to include international research and/or go further back in date so as to capture more data.

6.2.3 Hermeneutical exegesis: the synthesis and interpretive approach

Hermeneutics is the 'classical discipline concerned with the art of interpreting texts' (Gadamer, 1984: 146). The process of linguistic translation exemplifies hermeneutics well. In translation, let's say from English to French or vice versa, 'the original language of a text is replaced with another that yields a new understanding' (Gadamer, 1984: 345–351). In other words, once you have analyzed your data you will be replacing what you have synthesized from the data with your language and putting your interpretation on the literature. However, there is a danger that, in the absence of appropriate knowledge and skills, meaning can be lost in translation.

Exegesis is simply a term that defines the techniques for interpretation. It was initially developed to interpret biblical texts but has been extended to all textual data (Ramberg and Gjesdal, 2009). Gibbons (1987), cited in Boland et al. (2010), claims that exegesis enables those interpreting written texts to do the following:

- Recover the researcher's original meaning of the text
- Uncover hidden meaning that may have influenced the researcher's writing
- Discover meaning further than the context within which the writing was done.

This involves certain criteria against which the text is interpreted by iteration between criteria and text. Relevant to your research, the following are the four main criteria that characterize hermeneutic exegesis.

1 **Textual criticism** – This is establishing the accuracy of the text in order to obtain the best judgement about what is recorded in the text. In qualitative research studies, the key concerns are the accuracy of transcribed interviews. As you have learned in Chapter 5, it is not uncommon for this task to be undertaken by a person who is not involved in the

research. It is often undertaken by clerical staff who may not be familiar with the linguistic terms used in the interviews. Thus, there may be potential for errors in the transcripts. Here you may, where possible, examine the verbatim text quoted by the researchers to check for their accuracy. As for quantitative studies, it is not so much the textual context that is important, but the accuracy of methodological issues and its congruence with statistical representation of the findings.

2 **Historical criticism** – This is establishing how the historical context influences the meaning attached to the findings of research or what is written in grey literature. This also involves looking at what led to the research in the first place and what were the conditions and contexts under which the research studies were conducted. However, it is important to recognize at least two factors. First, the contexts may be different to your own practice settings. Secondly, as time changes so does the original understanding of the findings of research.

3 **Form criticism** – This is establishing how types of data (quantitative and/or qualitative) collected by the researcher and practices up to the time of writing and publication may affect the interpretation. In other words, form criticism entails tracking the steps of any research from its inception through to completion (see audit trail in Chapter 7) by examining how the context within which the research was conducted juxtaposes the researchers' philosophical positions. It is an important point to consider as this can ultimately influence the outcome of the research and what is published.

4 **Linguistic criticism** – This is establishing how the language employed in the text, in the form of its readability, affects the interpretation of data and subsequently the research outcome. If your selection of literature includes research that was conducted in countries other than English-speaking ones, then you may need to check for translation problems. Examples include text that may be mis-translated or simply mis-interpreted. In these cases, you may need to contact the researchers to obtain further clarification (see section 6.4.1 on missing data). (Adapted from Boland et al., 2010)

Student Activity 6.1 enables you to explore the above characteristics of hermeneutical exegesis.

================ **STUDENT ACTIVITY 6.1** ================

Using the same example of bowel cancer prevention and detection in Student Example 6.1, read and interrogate the findings from the five pieces of research. Go back and forth between these findings and the criteria that characterize hermeneutical exegesis. Answer the following questions:

- Are the methodological approaches of the five pieces of research congruent with their findings?
- Considering that bowel screening in the UK was conducted in 2000–2005, are the research findings within the contemporary context?

(Continued)

- What is your interpretation of Simon et al.'s (2011) research findings on the prevention of bowel cancer? (Take into account the current practices of healthcare professionals in providing information.)

Discuss your findings with another student or bring these to your next action learning set meeting.

The similarity between the two approaches of constant comparative analysis and hermeneutical exegesis is that they share an iterative characteristic and require as much iteration as necessary. The rationale behind this is to allow you to continue your analysis until you reach saturation point (Pidgeon and Henwood, 1996) – in other words, when you cannot see anything new in your data. While the constant comparative method of analysis allows for making comparisons, hermeneutical exegesis allows you to piece all the details together and make meaningful interpretations. Hermeneutical exegesis takes you beyond analysis and allows for interpretive synthesis, which culminates in the development of categories and themes. In order to identify themes, we must first know what a theme is. In the next section we outline the characteristics of themes.

6.3 What is a theme and the characteristics of a theme?

It is an unsound practice to refer to a theme in reports of research in an undefined and loose fashion in the absence of validating and supporting data. (DeSantis and Urgarriza, 2000: 367)

While there is consensus that a theme is the final outcome of data analysis, there seems to be no agreed definition of the term itself. In most research texts, terms such as 'concept', 'category' and 'theme' have been used interchangeably to convey the meaning of the term 'theme'. It is essential, therefore, to be clear about what we mean by themes. Thematic development is a critical stage in the accurate synthesis and meaningful interpretation of data. DeSantis and Ugarriza (2000) emphasize the importance of this process because it will bring rigour to your analysis and thus the outcome of your research will not be compromised.

In what follows we present a brief examination of the meaning of the term 'theme' to help you with this stage of your research project. In attempting to do so, we draw upon the work of Opler (1945) and Spradley (1979) within the discipline of anthropology. They assert that the development of themes is essentially a process of theorizing or theory formation that requires certain levels of abstraction. They describe the following characteristics of a theme:

- It is a cognitive principle
- It recurs in more than two domains
- It is tacit (it exists in a form that is not visible or accounted for and you need to search for it in order to make it visible)
- It denotes a position (either declared or implied)
- It has categories
- It links the categories (i.e. the relationship between words/phrases)
- It is a larger unit of thought that is made up of smaller components (from categories to overarching themes)
- It has a high degree of generalizability and it can be applied to numerous situations (such as its applicability to practice).

You will know that you have a theme if some of the elements described above are present. Student Activity 6.2 illustrates our point.

STUDENT ACTIVITY 6.2

Read the following explanation of a theme by Morse and Field (1995: 139–140):

> Themes are usually quite abstract and therefore do not immediately 'jump out' of the interview [*in your research this will be the literature-based data*], but may be more apparent if the researcher steps back and considers 'what are these folks trying to tell me?' [*in your research it will be what the literature-based data are trying to tell you*]. The theme may be beneath the surface of the interviews [i.e. *the literature-based data*], but once identified it will appear obvious.

Look again at the findings or data from the following five pieces of research:

Paper 1: Center et al. (2009) – worldwide trend analysis

The screening of bowel cancer has shown that early detection decreases mortality rates in developed countries by as much as 30% and the benefits of national and international bowel cancer screening programmes are irrefutable.

Paper 2: Goodyear et al. (2008) – retrospective trend analysis

Increased public awareness through the UK bowel cancer screening project in the West Midlands has positive impacts, such as attenuated emergency admissions, treatment and reduced mortality rates from bowel cancer.

(Continued)

Paper 3: Chapple et al. (2008) – qualitative interviews of the public

The uptake of the UK bowel cancer screening project in the form of faecal occult blood testing has been disappointing in some areas. More information on screening methods and people's experiences may increase participation by the public.

Paper 4: von Wagner et al. (2009) – national trend analysis

The average uptake of the UK bowel cancer screening project in the form of faecal occult blood testing has been low.

Paper 5: Simon et al. (2011) – qualitative interviews of healthcare professionals

Healthcare professionals believe that information about cancer should focus on improvements achieved through preventing and treating cancer.

The following categories were identified:

- Benefits of screening
- Uptake of screening was low/disappointing
- The public ask for more information on screening methods
- Healthcare professionals ask for more information on prevention and treatment.

Look beneath the surface of these categories and see what 'jumps out' at you. Can you identify one theme from the above categories? Does your theme fit some of the characteristics described above by Opler (1945) and Spradley (1979)?

Compare your findings with another student who has done the same activity and ask why you have arrived at similar or divergent themes?

6.3.1 Types of themes

When exploring research texts, we have come across the following classifications of themes:

1 **Categories or preset themes** – Taylor-Powell and Renner (2003: 3) claim that 'The researcher starts with pre-identified categories then searches the data that match these categories'. However, Buetow (2010) highlights a problem with this approach: you might limit yourself to a narrow perspective and miss other important categories that may contribute to salient conclusions. Therefore, it is important to keep an open mind at this stage of your analysis and synthesis.

2 **Emergent themes** – Here the researcher allows themes to emerge from the data (Taylor-Powell and Renner, 2003). However, it is important to realize that themes do not just leap out of your data and this process is not as straightforward as it seems. This requires a level of abstraction, in which rigorous intellectual processes are applied

to your data. This process is influenced by many factors, such as what the researcher seeks to find out, how the data is synthesized as well as the researcher's philosophical position (Srivastava and Hopwood, 2009). By being transparent with these processes, you can then convey confidence to the people who read your work. As categories emerge into themes, you (as the researcher) will begin to make interpretations. This is the stage of developing overarching themes.

3 **Overarching themes** – Here the researcher brings all emergent themes together into composite themes. In effect, it is like putting a jigsaw puzzle together; once completed it not only represents the whole but also shows how each piece relates to form the whole. Overarching themes are the findings of your comprehensive literature review.

Now we have defined what themes are, we guide you through the process of thematic development.

6.4 The process of developing themes

The purpose of developing themes is to provide a pathway to reaching an explanation about the research problem/topic under study. Since your comprehensive literature review is inclusive of papers from quantitative/qualitative research papers and grey literature, it is logical that your method of data analysis and synthesis needs to be pluralistic (Sandelowski et al., 2007). This is reinforced by Miles and Huberman (1994), who assert that all analysis has a reductive element to it. As stated earlier, you may need to start by using some form of simple quantification, such as counting. This is illustrated in Table 6.1 (see pages 128–129) below and Student Example 6.3 later on in this chapter.

Figure 6.2 describes thematic development using the iterative processes of analysis, synthesis and making an interpretation. It is based on the constant comparative method of analysis and hermeneutical exegesis.

From Figure 6.2 you can see that thematic development is a building-block process which may take a variety of steps. The process establishes relationships between categories, bringing them together into emergent themes and, finally, overarching themes. The processes of thematic development can be classified into three distinct stages:

1 An exploratory stage where data extraction occurs.
2 An analysis stage where data is interrogated and dialogued (i.e. the comparing and contrasting of what is in each piece of literature), as advocated in the constant comparative method of analysis.
3 A synthesis stage where the hermeneutical exegesis approach is applied to show how meaning is created through rigorous process, exemplified by cross-referencing your interpretation of yourself as a researcher and with other reliable sources.

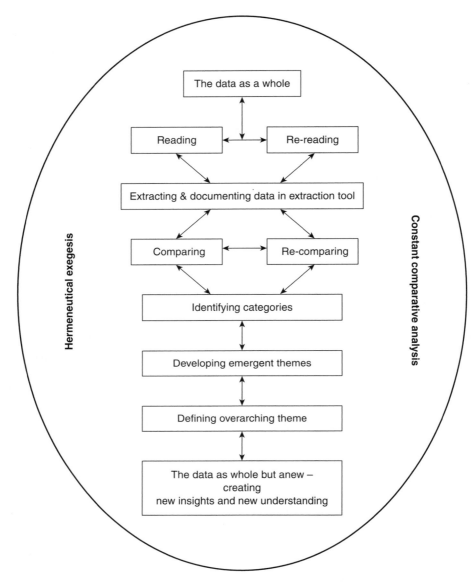

Figure 6.2 Thematic development using the processes of analysis and synthesis based on the principles of constant comparative methods of analysis and hermeneutical exegesis (adapted from Boland et al., 2010)

6.4.1 The exploratory stage

At the start of the exploratory stage, you will have decided on a set of evaluative criteria against which to analyze the selected literature, and devised a data extraction/summary table in readiness for data entry. This stage is descriptive but very important. As discussed in Chapter 5, this entails stripping the data, to unravel and examine the data in its simplest form (Clough and Nutbrown, 2000). It involves reading and re-reading, comparing and contrasting data with the set of evaluative criteria that you have devised. This is synonymous with the 'back and forth' process of constant comparative analysis (Strauss and Corbin, 1994). The purpose of this process is to ensure that you do not miss any data or important categories (Ryan and Bernard, 2003), so that no stone is left unturned. You may also need to search for missing data as these can influence the conclusions that you draw from your synthesis and interpretation (Cooper, 2010). In some cases of quantitative research, Cooper (2010) explains that missing data, such as incomplete statistical information, is used by researchers to support or reject hypotheses. This kind of omission may indicate a number of things, including that 'the researcher may choose not to include the exact results of statistical tests and may simply report that there was no statistical significance' (Cooper, 2010: 105). This is often found in many research reports. Other examples of missing data may be related to the design of the study, such as the representativeness of the sample, the setting of the study, such as the hospital or community settings, and national or international contexts (Cooper, 2010). Missing data can also be present in published qualitative research reports. The following Student Example 6.2 illustrates missing data at the analysis and synthesis stage of the research process.

Student Example 6.2   Missing data in a piece of qualitative research

The following are excerpts from a qualitative research conducted in Norway:

A. Lyberg and E. Severinsson (2010) 'Fear of childbirth: mothers' experiences of team-midwifery care – a follow-up study', Journal of Nursing Management, 18(4), 383–390.

Aim: The aim of this study was to illuminate mothers' fear of childbirth and their experiences of the team-midwifery care model during pregnancy, childbirth and the postnatal period.

Methods: This hermeneutic study comprised interviews with 13 women, which were audio-taped and transcribed verbatim, after which interpretative content analysis was performed. Ethical approval was granted.

Sample: The inclusion criterion was that the women had attended the intervention and had had at least three individual consultations with one of the

(Continued)

four midwives on the team before giving birth. The women ranged in age from 25 to 37 years. Seven reported that they had had negative experiences of their first childbirth, three of whom had undergone an emergency caesarean section and two had complications requiring vacuum extraction. Before the intervention, four of the women had no children, six had one child, two had two and one had three children.

Results: The findings revealed one main theme: '*The woman's right to ownership of the pregnancy, childbirth and postnatal care as a means of maintaining dignity*' and three other themes: '*Being aware of barriers and reasons for fear*'; '*Being prepared for childbirth*' and '*Being confirmed and treated with dignity by the midwife*'. Each theme contained several sub-themes.

In order to illustrate our point on missing data, we have also included the following extract from the journal article's 'Results' section:

Being prepared for childbirth

In this theme, the women reported their need to be involved as well as supervised by a familiar midwife. One woman stated her feelings about the *body-in-labour*:

'I was not physically afraid, I did not fear the pain itself, no I was afraid of the routines, the possibility of hands in my body to inspect whether I was "open" [ready for] birth, without involving me in the decision. Giving birth is a situation where you feel vulnerable and at the mercy of someone you might not know at all.'

Another woman described her feelings about her body-in-labour as *being intruded upon*:

'You are so exposed and naked when giving birth. It is the most private and intimate unpleasant situation you will ever experience.'

Some of the women reported that they *wanted to know the midwife very well* and have an individual *care and birth plan* for pregnancy and childbirth:

'The midwife gave me a lot of information and supervised me with regard to pregnancy and birth. I could not have managed the postpartum period without that. My baby cried a great deal and was not satisfied with anything or anybody but me for four months – it was very hard for me.'

For the theme '*Being prepared for childbirth*' there were three sub-themes. These are italicized in the text above. As you can see, there is one verbatim quote from the participants to support each sub-theme. However, some important facts, which would have impacted on the researchers' interpretation of the data, are missing. These are:

1 The number of quotations used to support each sub-theme.
2 The sample characteristics, such as the number of births and previous experience (characteristics that were not related to the verbatim quotations), may impact on the women's feelings of being prepared for childbirth.

All-in-all, this places doubts on the validity or trustworthiness of the findings as the interpretation of the themes extracted from the interviews with the women were not made explicit. Despite the missing data, this research has given adequate background information regarding the maternity services in Norway. There was transparency in some stages of the research process (such as access to participants, the conduct of the interviews, the procedure of content analysis), which contributed to the rigour of the research findings.

However, missing data are more than methodological concerns; they may also be ethical ones, particularly if they relate to honesty and accountability, as discussed in Chapter 5. Missing data may jeopardize the analysis and synthesis of your selected literature. Cooper (2010: 106–107) identifies several ways of dealing with missing data:

- You can contact the researcher for further information
- You can examine other documents that describe the reported study to obtain the missing information (this may be a dissertation or thesis from which the published study originates).

On completing the exploratory stage, you will now have a display of the data you have extracted. Table 6.1 is an example of a completed data extraction table based on data extracted from seven pieces of literature on the role of the midwife in establishing relationships with clients.

6.4.2 The analysis stage

In this section the building-block principle of thematic development is further explored. In our experience, students have found this stage challenging, so do make sure you spend sufficient time on this process. Once you have a documented display of the preliminary findings of your analysis you are in a position to begin the identification of categories.

Before you start this stage we recommend that you complete Student Activity 6.3.

Table 6.1 Exemplar of a completed data extraction table – 'the role of the midwife in establishing relationships with clients'

Date	Author/ researcher	Philosophical basis	Research question	Methodology	Sample	Data collection	Data analysis	Findings	Conclusions
Paper 1 Harvey et al. (2002)	5 Canadian researchers: 3 midwives, 1 doctor and 1 statistician	Quantitative (positivism)	2 hypotheses: more women 1. are satisfied 2. have positive attitude regarding midwife care	Randomized controlled trial	194 women experimental group (midwife care) and control group (doctor care)	3 satisfaction questionnaires (LADSI, ADLE & SSQ) at predetermined intervals	Statistical analysis using SPSS	Women in midwife group had greater satisfaction and more positive experience	Dated study possible changes in Canadian healthcare system in last decade Good design and well executed
Paper 2 Symon et al. (2011)	5 British researchers: 2 with nursing or midwifery background; 1 statistician	Quantitative (positivism)	Examine views & experiences of environment, service provision and care	Postal survey	515 mothers and same birth partners from 6 midwife-led and 3 obstetric-led units	Satisfaction questionnaire given to mother and birth partners separately 8 days postnatal	Statistical analysis using SPSS	Mothers and partners were both positive; mothers rated midwifery care and birth surroundings better than doctor-led units	Disproportionate sample from midwife versus doctor-led units Focus on partners as well as mothers
Paper 3 Fereday et al. (2009)	5 Australian researchers: 3 with nursing or midwifery background	Mixed methodology (positivism and interpretivism)	Aim to determine women's satisfaction with MGP model of care	Postal survey with both closed and open questions	84 women in Midwife Group Practice (MGP)	Self-developed satisfaction questionnaire over 3-month antenatal period	Statistical analysis likert scale questions; content analysis of open questions	Women satisfied with MGP care; continuity, accessibility and attributes of midwives add to positive scores	Small sample Triangulation of findings add rigour to study
Paper 4 Hildingsson et al. (2011)	3 Swedish researchers: all researchers linked to university in Sweden	Quantitative (positivism)	Aim to identify fathers' experiences of normal birth and factors related to midwife care	Part of a longitudinal survey	595 fathers present at birth, women under care of midwife	Questionnaire given mid-pregnancy and again after birth	Statistical analysis of likert questions using SPSS	82% of fathers had positive experiences: midwife presence, support and information giving	Fathers only in one particular region of Sweden Maternity care system in Sweden briefly elaborated

Date	Author/ researcher	Philosophical basis	Research question	Methodology	Sample	Data collection	Data analysis	Findings	Conclusions
Paper 5 McCourt (2006)	1 English researcher: researcher in midwifery practice	Qualitative (interpretivism)	Aim to explore interaction of women and midwives with caseload model	Not stated	40 interactions of midwives and pregnant mothers in hospital, GP clinic and home	Taped interviews and observational notes	Content analysis using structured and qualitative approaches	International patterns in midwifery caseload model of care: less hierarchical, more conversational, offered more information, choice and control	Hawthorne effect on performance of midwives and reaction of mothers Data source triangulation boost rigour
Paper 6 Raine et al. (2010)	5 English researchers: 2 researchers, 1 consultant midwife and 2 psychologists	Qualitative (interpretivism)	4 stated aims focusing on the elements of communication that need to be tackled	Not stated	30 pregnant women communication experiences in antenatal period	Focus group and semi-structured interviews	Thematic analysis	Good communication: empathetic style, openness to questions, time to talk, text reminders of appointments Poor communication: insufficient information and discussion, discourteous style	London area only Focused on both good and bad communications; some good recommendations, such as training, more integration with GPs and use of technologies
Paper 7 Royal College of Obstetricians and Gynaecologists (2008)	Royal College of Obstetricians and Gynaecologists	Government report (unspecified)	Not relevant	Not relevant	Based on 50 documents by government and maternity organizations	Not relevant	Not relevant	Standard 22: communication	Clear guidelines on high-quality care and self-audit

To embark on this exercise, have your research question/statement at hand.

Complete your data extraction or summary table and make sure you are familiar with the data (literature findings). Then ask what you will need from the data in your data extraction or summary table to answer your research question/statement.

Re-examine your philosophical position at this stage of your research and check if it has changed since completing Student Activity 2.4 in Chapter 2. What would be the intended application to practice?

Keep your answers to this activity as you will find it useful to refer to it later in the final stage of your synthesis.

Thematic development begins with comparing and contrasting, i.e. looking for similarities and differences. A number of terms have been used to define this process. Examples include categorizing and coding. In this chapter we use the term 'categorizing' as the starting point. It is a stringent and painstaking process as it is necessary to 'go back and forth' to your data while maintaining the interrogation and dialogue with the data (as advocated in the principles of constant comparative analysis). By doing this, the important categories are not missed.

Developing categories involves a combination of deductive and inductive approaches. It starts with the deductive approach, where you will be organizing your categories by using your own words or descriptions to form key phrases. The following steps will help you develop categories:

- Search the data for key phrases or ideas
- Count the frequency with which these key phrases or ideas recur across the literature
- Look for similarities and differences in key phrases or ideas
- Ask how similar they are (similar characteristics)
- Ask how key phrases differ from each other (conflicting characteristics). Conflicting characteristics, as the term implies, will provide you with a sound basis for recommending future research.

To complement the above steps, we suggest you use Buetow's (2010: 124) coding system, which looks at the importance of different types of categories or key phrases. These categories are:

1 Highly important and recurrent categories or key phrases. These can be identified by counting how often a category or key phrase appears in and across all the papers.
2 Highly important but not recurrent categories or key phrases. These can be identified by noting their significance to your research question/statement.
3 Not highly important but recurrent categories or key phrases.

Looking for categories or key phrases entails finding the above characteristics in your data. This will require you to cross-check the literature using a systematic approach. You may choose to display how you arrive at the themes in a matrix by colour coding or using different type styles for each category or key phrase. The exemplar in Table 6.2 suggests ways to make this process manageable and transparent, and opens the possibility for meaningful interpretation that can improve your understanding of literature-based data.

It is important to note that the iterative processes of counting the frequency of categories and searching the data to support these categories may be seen as analogous to having a hypothesis and then setting out to test it. However, the process of iteration takes you beyond the positivist deductive paradigm to also situate your analysis in the interpretivist inductive paradigm. This demonstrates the movement between paradigms and is in keeping with the pluralistic nature of the comprehensive literature review methodology. Often these two paradigms are used to describe competing philosophical views about the nature of knowledge in the social world and the ways in which social reality should be studied (Patton, 1990; Guba and Lincoln, 1994). But as you may find both paradigms, although divergent in their orientation, may in fact complement each other in informing the design of your comprehensive review.

The next stage is the final process of thematic development and it continues with the iterative process as well as the pluralistic principle used with all the other stages.

6.4.3 The synthesis stage

Synthesis is a crucial stage of your research project and it is an aspect that has often been weak in the way it is undertaken. It is about bringing your analyzed data into a meaningful whole by utilizing a higher level of abstraction. The purpose is to develop emergent themes into overarching themes. In doing so, you are interpreting the findings from your research with new insight and in a more coherent way. This will help you make sense of the research problem that you set out to solve in the first instance (Strike and Posner, 1983; Paterson et al., 2001). It is also important to show how your philosophical position has shaped your synthesis by taking responsibility for your findings so as to demonstrate reflexivity and compliance with the ethical principles of integrity, transparency and accountability.

The synthesis process requires replacing what you have found in your data with a new language by putting your own interpretation on the findings. In bringing together all the components you have separated out back into a whole, it is important to remember that it is not and cannot be the same whole. Here you need to ask yourself, 'What does this all mean to my research?' To answer

Table 6.2 Example of thematic development – 'the role of the midwife in establishing relationships with clients'

	Categories or key phrases	Frequency of categories () = paper no.	Similar characteristics (see symbols)	Conflicting characteristics	Categories	Relationship of categories (see symbols)	Emergent themes	Overarching themes
Paper 1 Harvey et al. (2002)	*In favour of **midwife-led care (MLC)**	MLC (1,2&3)	√	none	**Midwife-led**	§	Midwife-led care increases continuity	Relationships with clients are promoted by increased continuity
Paper 2 Symon et al. (2011)	*In favour of **MLC** *Fathers rated better birth surroundings	Birth surroundings (2)	√	none				
Paper 3 Fereday et al. (2008)	*Continuity of care in **midwife-care model = MLC** *Accessibility *Positive attributes of midwives	Continuity (3) Midwife attributes & support (3&4)	√ Φ	none	Continuity Accessibility	§	Continuity, presence and accessibility	Relationships with clients are promoted by midwife presence & accessibility
Paper 4 Hildingsson et al. (2011)	*Fathers rated positively of midwife support, presence and information giving	Presence & accessibility (3&4)	Φ	none	Presence	§		

	Categories or key phrases	Frequency of categories ( ) = paper no.	Similar characteristics (see symbols)	Conflicting characteristics	Categories	Relationship of categories (see symbols)	Emergent themes	Overarching themes
Paper 5 McCourt (2006)	***More conversational and less hierarchical form of communication** *Greater information, choice and control	Information giving (4,5&7) Choice (5) Control (5)	Σ	none	Information giving	Ж		Relationships with clients are promoted by giving clients choice of information
Paper 6 Raine et al. (2010)	*__Empathetic conversational style__ *OPENNESS TO QUESTIONS *Text messaging as appointment reminders	__Style of conversation: effective, sensitive&__ __conversational__ (5,6&7) OPEN TO QUESTIONS (6)	Σ Φ	none	**Conversational** **style** **(empathetic,** **sensitive)**	®	Giving the choice of information	
Paper 7 Maternity Care Report (2008)	*Aspect of choice and time to reflect on information *Information communicated in an __effective & sensitive__ __manner__ *Effective systems of communication	Choice (5&7) Time to reflect (7) Systems of communication e.g. text messaging (6&7)	Σ	none	Choice of information Effective systems of communication	Ж ®	Effective style and systems of communication	Relationships with clients are promoted by styles and systems of communication

this question requires you to return to the principle of hermeneutical exegesis, which enables you to do the following:

- Enter into the different worlds of the researchers of the studies you have examined
- Lay each set of findings bare and see the contribution that each has made to the whole, i.e. your research problem/topic
- Integrate your own philosophical position with that of the researchers of the studies you have examined.

In other words, the above defines a process of bringing together different perspectives. This is akin to Gadamer's notion of fusion of horizons (1984) which he defined as a process of interpreting a text (in your case, literature-based data). In order to understand the concept of 'fusion of horizons' and how to apply it to the art of interpretation you need to understand the key ideas that underpin it. Fusion is another term for synthesis; the tenets of 'fusion of horizons' are not only about meaning or knowledge but, more importantly, they are about understanding what shapes how we create meaning or knowledge. Horizon is a term that defines the entirety of our life world and encapsulates our history and culture. Gadamer (1984) asserts that the fusion of horizons recognizes the interplay and interdependence of our history and culture. In the context of our professional world, this is akin to the scope of our practice and the utilization of interpreted evidence to inform our practice. The key factors shaping the process of interpretation can be summed up as our ontological and epistemological perspectives or horizons. As you have learned in Chapter 2, researchers as well as those being researched bring different ontological and epistemological horizons to their research. In other words, research is designed, conducted, analyzed and reported within different horizons. Therefore, it is important to recognize that literature-based data are not exempt from these horizons, as the process of interpretation is vital in ensuring that your findings reflect the interplay between the different horizons. In your comprehensive literature review, this calls for the engagement of your own horizon with the text (literature-based data). Gadamer (1984) claimed that one must embrace other horizons when interpreting data; in so doing, we expand our understanding and increase our knowledge of the subject of inquiry. To unravel this you may find Figure 6.3 helpful. We have also added the disciplinary or professional context as another horizon, as the linkage you will make between your research and the wider perspectives of each of the other horizons will help to illuminate larger issues about the findings of your research.

Student Example 6.3 illustrates the process of thematic development and the notion of Gadamer's fusion of horizons (1984).

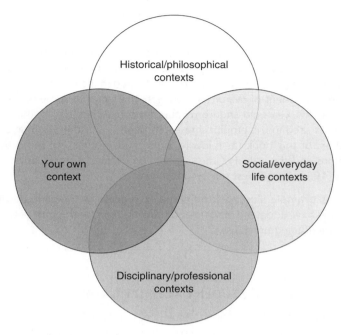

Historical/philosophical
contexts

Your own
context

Social/everyday
life contexts

Disciplinary/professional
contexts

Figure 6.3 Fusion of horizons

Student Example 6.3 **Moving from categories to emergent themes to overarching themes in the process of thematic development**

Here we are referring to the example of thematic development in Table 6.2 on the subject of 'The role of the midwife in establishing relationships with clients'.

You will have noted that the moving from categories to emergent themes involved examples of two vital processes from opposing paradigmatic standpoints:

1 **Counting** (using the positivist paradigm) – The frequency of categories was noted from each of the seven chosen pieces of literature, 'Midwife-led care' and 'Information giving' being the most frequently occurring categories.
2 **Constant comparison** (using the interpretivist paradigm) – The interpretation of the categories and their meaning enabled us to see relationships in the form of similarities. This allowed us to start clustering the categories to form emerging themes. For example, 'Midwife-led care and continuity', 'Continuity, presence and accessibility' were interpreted to be similar. In this example, there were no conflicting characteristics in the identified categories; if these were present, we would need to go back and re-examine and re-interpret our findings. Hence, it is an iterative process.

(Continued)

(Continued)

As *emergent themes* were formed, we delved into the socio-cultural and historical context of each piece of literature analyzed, as well as the philosophical position of the researchers and our own, which ultimately helped in the hermeneutical interpretation and development of *overarching themes*. The fact that some of the literature was more than five years old and from countries other than the UK, the contrasting methodologies used in the empirical research papers, and the personal experience of the authors of this book (as midwife, nurse and mother), all bring to bear on interpretations and the arrival of the overarching themes. This is Gadamer's fusion of horizons (1984) in its fullest sense.

We hope this example illustrates the complex process of thematic development. Make sure you have adequate reading and thinking time for this part of the research process (as mentioned previously).

STUDENT ACTIVITY 6.4

Now refer to your answers from Student Activity 6.3 and begin to construct a table (as in Table 6.2). Sometimes, you need to stand back and look at the findings from the literature with 'fresh' eyes, to reflect on your own preliminary interpretations and bring these to your action learning sets so as to gain a better insight on the topic before you arrive at the final product.

To summarize, synthesis involves putting your overarching themes within the broader context of your research. This helps you to distinguish the context within which empirical research was conducted or the context within which policy was formulated (as in non-empirical research). In essence, it is a synergistic process that 'involves some degree of conceptual innovation, or employment of concepts not found in the characteristics of the part' (Strike and Posner, 1983: 346).

The four horizons identified in the model above may enable you to bring your own innovation and creativity to your research. It may also provide 'valuable insights about how research has been conducted and where' (Paterson et al., 2001: 87). As well as enabling you to blend your own horizon with the wider contexts stated above, this model provides a way for you to demonstrate their collective relevance in arriving at new insights. Synthesis therefore entails looking at all the horizons, fusing them together to gain a new perspective on the subject of study (Boote and Beile, 2005; Cooper, 2010).

In essence, synthesis enables you, through the interpretive process of hermeneutical exegesis, to make recommendations that are significant, which will assist in the further development of your profession. A pitfall of many syntheses is that recommendations for further research are not based on rigorous, systematic and iterative processes. This may indicate that the data has not been fully utilized (Weed, 2005). In the next chapter we guide you through the presentation and discussion of findings from your synthesis.

End-of-Chapter Learning Points

We hope that you have found this chapter helpful in understanding the processes involved in thematic development. The following are some of the key points highlighted in this chapter:

1 Undertaking analysis and synthesis of data requires a systematic and transparent approach.
2 There are discrete stages in thematic development: the exploratory stage, the analysis stage and the synthesis stage.
3 In order to be clear about how to identify themes we also need to be clear about what we mean by the term 'theme'. DeSantis and Urgarriza (2000: 367) remind us that 'it is unsound practice to refer to a theme in reports of research in an undefined and loose fashion in the absence of validating and supporting data'.
4 The theoretical framework of constant comparative analysis and hermeneutical exegesis enables a more discursive approach in thematic development. It also enables the achievement of a higher level of intellectual skills.
5 Above all, your voice and reflexivity are important as they show creativity and independent thinking in your development as an innovative thinker.
6 In conducting your comprehensive literature review, you will develop intellectual skills, an understanding of research and the capacity to pursue research as a career later on if you wish to.

References

On bowel cancer

Center, M.M., Jemal, A., Smith, R.A. and Ward E. (2009) 'Worldwide variations in colorectal cancer', *CA: A Cancer Journal for Clinicians*, 59(6), 366–378.
Chapple, A., Ziebland, S., Hewitson, P. and McPherson, A. (2008) 'What affects the uptake of screening for bowel cancer using a faecal occult blood test (FOBt): a qualitative study', *Social Science & Medicine*, 66(12), 2425–2435.
Goodyear, S.J., Leung, E., Menon, A., Pedamallu, S., William, N. and Wong, L.S. (2008) 'The effects of population-based faecal occult blood test screening upon emergency colorectal cancer admissions in Coventry and north Warwickshire', *Gut*, 57, 218–222.

Simon, A.E., Wardle, J. and Miles, A. (2011) 'Is it time to change the stereotype of cancer: the expert view?', *Cancer Causes Control*, 22, 135–140.

von Wagner, C., Good, A., Wright, D., Rachet, B., Obichere, A., Bloom, S. and Wardle, J. (2009) 'Inequalities in colorectal cancer screening participation in the first round of the national screening programme in England', *British Journal of Cancer*, 101, S60–S63.

On midwifery care

Fereday, J., Collins, C., Turnbull, D. and Pincombe, J. (2009) 'An evaluation of midwifery group practice. Part II: women's satisfaction', *Women and Birth*, 22(1), 11–16.

Harvey, S., Rach, D., Stainton, M.C., Jarrell, J. and Brant, R. (2002) 'Evaluation of satisfaction with midwifery care', *Midwifery*, 18(4), 260–267.

Hildingsson, I., Cederlof, L. and Widén, S. (2011) 'Fathers' birth experience in relation to midwifery care', *Women and Birth*, 24(3), 129–136.

McCourt, C. (2006) 'Supporting choice and control? Communication and interaction between midwives and women at the antenatal booking visit', *Social Science and Medicine*, 62(6), 1307–1318.

Raine, R., Cartwright, M., Richens, Y., Mahamed, Z. and Smith, D. (2010) 'A qualitative study of women's experiences of communication in antenatal care: identifying areas for action', *Maternal and Child Health Journal*, 14(4), 590–599.

Royal College of Obstetricians and Gynaecologists (2008) *Standards for Maternity Care: Report of a Working Party*. London: RCOG Press. Available at: www.rcog.org.uk/files/rcog-corp/uploaded-files/WPRMaternityStandards2008.pdf (accessed on 4 July 2012).

Symon, A.G., Dugard, P., Butchart, M., Carr, V. and Paul, J. (2011) 'Care and environment in midwife-led and obstetric-led units: a comparison of mothers' and birth partners' perceptions', *Midwifery*, 27(6), 880–886.

On defining and identifying themes

Buetow, S. (2010) 'Thematic analysis and its reconceptualisation as "saliency analysis"', *Journal of Health Services Research and Policy*, 15(2), 123–125.

DeSantis, L. and Ugarriza, D.N. (2000) 'The concept of themes as used in qualitative nursing research', *Western Journal of Nursing*, 22, 331.

Opler, M.E. (1945) 'Themes as dynamic forces in culture', *American Journal of Sociology*, 51(3), 198–206.

Ryan, G.W. and Bernard, H.R. (2003) 'Techniques to identify themes', *Field Methods*, 15(1), 85–109.

Spradley, J.P. (1979) *The Ethnographic Interview*. New York: Holt, Rhinehart & Winston.

On research and method of data analysis and synthesis

Boland, R.J., Newman, M. and Pentland, B.T. (2010) 'Hermeneutical exegesis in information system design and use', *Information and Organisation*, 20(1020), 1–20.

Boote, D.N. and Beile, P. (2005) 'Scholars before researchers: on the centrality of the dissertation literature review in research preparation', *Educational Researcher*, 34(6), 3–15.

Charmaz, K. (2006) *Constructing Grounded Theory*. Thousand Oaks, CA: Sage.

Clough, P. and Nutbrown, C. (2000) *A Student's Guide to Methodology*. London: Sage.

Cooper, H. (2010) *Research Synthesis and Meta-Analysis*. Thousand Oaks, CA: Sage.

Gadamer, H.G. (1984) *Truth and Method*. New York: Crossroads.

Glaser, B.G. (1978) *Theoretical Sensitivity: Advances in the Methodology of Grounded Theory*. Mill Valley, CA: Sociology Press.

Glaser, B.G. (1992) *Emergence vs. Forcing: Basics of Grounded Theory Analysis*. Mill Valley, CA: Sociology Press.

Glaser, B.G. and Strauss, A. (1967) *The Discovery of Grounded Theory*. Chicago, IL: Aldine.

Guba, E.G. and Lincoln, Y.S. (1994) 'Competing paradigms in qualitative research', in N.K. Denzin and Y.S. Lincoln (eds), *Handbook of Qualitative Research*. London: Sage.

Miles, M.B. and Huberman, A.M. (1994) *Qualitative Data Analysis*. Thousand Oaks, CA: Sage.

Morse, J.M. and Field, P.A. (1995) *Qualitative Research Methods for Health Professionals* (2nd edn). Thousand Oaks, CA: Sage.

Oxford Dictionaries (1990) *Oxford Dictionary of English*. Oxford: Oxford University Press.

Paterson, B.L., Thorne, E.S., Cannan, C. and Jillings, C. (2001) *Meta-Study of Qualitative Health Research: A Practical Guide to Meta-Analysis and Meta-Synthesis*. Thousand Oaks, CA: Sage.

Patton, M. (1990) *Qualitative Evaluation and Research Methods*. Beverly Hills, CA: Sage.

Pidgeon, N. and Henwood, K. (1996) 'Grounded theory: practical implementation', in J.T.E. Richardson (ed.), *Handbook of Qualitative Research Methods for Psychology and the Social Sciences*. Leicester: BPS Books.

Popay, J. (2006) Moving beyond Effectiveness in Evidence Synthesis: *Methodological Issues in the Synthesis of Diverse Sources of Evidence*. London: National Institute for Health and Clinical Excellence. Available at: www.publichealth.nice.org.uk.

Ramberg, B. and Gjesdal, K. (2009) 'Hermeneutics', in N.Z. Edward (eds), *The Stanford Encyclopedia of Philosophy*. Stanford, CA: The Metaphysics Research Lab.

Sandelowski, M., Barroso, J. and Voils, I.C. (2007) 'Using qualitative metasummary to synthesize qualitative and quantitative descriptive findings', *Research in Nursing and Health*, 30(1), 99–111.

Srivastava, P. and Hopwood, N. (2009) 'A practical iterative framework for qualitative data analysis', *International Journal of Qualitative Methods*, 8(1), 76–84.

Strauss, A. and Corbin, J. (1994) 'Grounded theory methodology: an overview', in N.K. Denzin and Y.S. Lincoln (eds), *Handbook of Qualitative Research*. Thousand Oaks, CA: Sage.

Strike, K. and Posner, G. (1983) 'Types of synthesis and their criteria', in A.W. Spencer and L.J. Reed (eds), *Knowledge, Structure and Use*. Philadelphia, PA: Temple University Press.

Taylor-Powell, E. and Renner, M. (2003) *Analyzing Qualitative Data: Programme Development and Evaluation*. Madison: University of Wisconsin-Extension. Available at: www.learning-store.uwex.edu/assets/pdfs/g3658-12.pdf (accessed 4 July 2012).

Weed, M. (2005) 'Meta interpretation: a method for the interpretative synthesis of qualitative research', *Forum Qualitative Social Research,* 6(1) [online article], www.qualitative-research.net/index.php/fqs/article/view/508/1096 (accessed 9 February 2012).

Whittemore, R. and Knafl, K. (2005) 'The integrative review: updated methodology', *Journal of Advanced Nursing*, 52(5), 546–553.

SEVEN

Presentation and Discussion of Findings

Aim and objectives

The aim of this chapter is to assist you in presenting your findings and discussing the results of your comprehensive literature review in a logical manner. By the end of the chapter you will be able to:

- Present the findings by providing an initial overview followed by summaries of findings from empirical and non-empirical literature
- Discuss the methodological rigour of each piece of literature as a continuous thread and explain how this boosts the rigour of your comprehensive literature review
- Compare other ways of increasing the rigour of your comprehensive literature review
- Recognize the strengths and limitations of your comprehensive literature review
- Identify the need for generalization or transferability of findings so as to make recommendations for practice, education and further research.

7.1 Introduction

Chapter 5 took you through the analysis process and culminated with the critical findings from all the literature you have scrutinized. These findings are equivalent to raw data collected in empirical research. They are treated in just the same way as these are summarized in diagrammatic format. In the case of the comprehensive literature review methodology, the diagrams are in form of data extraction (or summary) tables and these are placed in your appendices. The next stage, discussed in Chapter 6, is the process of analysis and synthesis, which is vital in the identification and formulation of themes. Here you are working in a pluralistic manner, both deductively and inductively, so that categories emerge from your data from which these overarching themes are formulated. This chapter moves the research process on further. It is broken down into two stages:

1 Presenting the findings by discussing the summary data from your data extraction tables.
2 Discussing the findings by focusing on one theme at a time.

7.2 Presenting the findings

This section explains how to present and describe the findings from your data. You need to be aware that the findings generated are vast as a large amount of literature may be scrutinized and analyzed. It is impossible to present the findings from individual pieces of literature, so there are ways of grouping them together to create order and sense in your discussion. There are no fixed rules as to how this is done. The following is a suggested format, which is dependent on the type of literature selected for your comprehensive literature review:

- Overview of your findings
- Summary of quantitative research findings
- Summary of qualitative research findings
- Summary of findings from grey literature

(As the number of research papers using mixed methodology tend to be small, the summary of these can be amalgamated with the quantitative or qualitative research findings – see Student Example 7.2.)

7.2.1 Overview of your findings

A brief overview of your findings can be given by highlighting some of the following key points:

- Range of dates
- UK versus international literature
- Empirical versus non-empirical literature
- Quantitative versus qualitative literature
- Audits versus governmental reports.

This can be displayed as a table in your main text. You can comment on the spread of literature in relation to the possible abundance or lack of literature in certain areas. You can also comment on how this has affected the quality of your research.

In order to demonstrate your understanding of how different literature contributed to the findings of your comprehensive literature review and ultimately the generation of categories and themes, there needs to be a discussion based around the three main groups of literature: quantitative research, qualitative research and grey literature (plus a possible fourth group of mixed methodology research). The next few sections demonstrate how this is done.

7.2.2 Summary of quantitative research findings

In your selected pieces of empirical literature you may have analyzed some quantitative research. As mentioned before, the findings from your analysis are summarized in data extraction or summary tables and placed in the appendix of your research report. Student Example 7.1 illustrates how you can comment on your quantitative research findings. As this example is fictitious, the authors' names and date of publication are not quoted in the text.

Student Example 7.1   Summarizing findings from three quantitative papers

Research Statement 1: *There are differences between the public and health-care professionals in their viewpoints on the prevention and detection of bowel cancer.*

There are three quantitative research papers all utilizing survey methodology. The authors are nurses and statisticians. One of the papers is from Canada, whereas the other two are from the UK. The Canadian paper and one of the UK papers are cross-sectional surveys, whereas the remaining one is a longitudinal survey gathering data over a period of four years. All three research projects collected data using questionnaires, except for the Canadian one where the researchers followed up with face-to-face interviews of volunteer participants (around 10% of the sample). The findings from all three pieces of research unanimously supported the screening of bowel cancer by testing for faecal occult blood (FOB). However, the public's and healthcare professionals' views differ in relation to how funds should be used for the prevention and detection of bowel cancer.

In this example, the research statement relates to three pieces of quantitative research. We have illustrated how you can summarize the findings from quantitative research papers by commenting on the authors, sources of publications, research designs, methods of data collection and, lastly, a brief overview of the findings.

You will have also noticed that we have avoided making comments on the quality of the research papers as this can be left until you discuss the findings (see section 7.3).

7.2.3 Summary of qualitative research findings

The findings from the analyzed qualitative research papers (summarized in your data extraction or summary tables) are discussed in the same way as the quantitative research findings. In Student Example 7.2, findings from eight qualitative research papers and two papers utilizing mixed methodology are discussed together, as there are two research questions that relate to these ten empirical studies. Again, the example is fictitious so the authors' surnames and years are not quoted in the text.

Student Example 7.2   Summarizing findings from eight qualitative papers and two using mixed methodologies

Research Question 1: *How is bowel cancer prevented and detected?*

Research Question 2: *How do the public and professionals feel about the way bowel cancer is prevented and detected?*

There are eight qualitative research papers. Four are international research papers and four are from the UK. Six of the papers utilized a phenomeno-logical approach and data were collected from both public and healthcare professionals using face-to-face and focus group interviews. The remaining two qualitative papers did not claim to use any particular qualitative research methodologies. These two pieces of research utilized face-to-face interview techniques. The two papers with mixed methodologies were conducted in the USA; they utilized a mixture of surveys and focus group interviews to gather data from the public and from healthcare professionals. All ten pieces of research were conducted by healthcare professionals, mostly specialist cancer nurses, but two papers from the UK also involved doctors. The findings were mixed regarding the detection of bowel cancer. The public identified the lack of information on government screening initiatives, such as the FOB screening, as the main cause of missed diagnosis. Healthcare professionals, on the other hand, claimed that resources were wasted on screening for bowel cancer and felt that more emphasis should be placed on prevention. Specialist cancer nurses were aware of the importance of prevention, but their role was predominantly in the detection and treatment of bowel cancer. Healthcare professionals surveyed felt that the government should place more emphasis on lifestyle changes as preventative measures against bowel cancer.

In this example, we have chosen to comment on the qualitative and mixed method-ology research papers at the same time. Here we focused on the authors' professional status, the sources of publications in relation to which country they originated from, the research designs, sample groups and methods of data collection. Lastly, the find-ings from all ten papers were summarized with the two research questions in mind.

Again, you will have noticed that we have avoided comments on the quality of the research papers as this can be left until you discuss the findings (see section 7.3).

7.2.4 Summary of findings from grey (non-empirical) literature

In this section, the findings from grey literature, such as government reports and audits, are summarized. These will have been scrutinized and analyzed in the same way as empirical literature. Please refer to the suggested criteria mentioned in section 5.4 of Chapter 5 for critiquing grey literature.

STUDENT ACTIVITY 7.1

Consider the following research statement:

> **Research Statement 2**: *There are varying degrees of success in local and government strategies in preventing and detecting bowel cancer.*

Refer to the following pieces of grey literature:

- Department of Health (2011) *Improving Outcomes: A Strategy for Cancer.* London: HMSO (a government document published in January 2011), www.dh.gov.uk/en/Publicationsandstatistics/Publications/PublicationsPolicyAndGuidance/DH_123371
- Sussex Cancer Network (2010) *National Awareness and Early Diagnosis Initiative: Baseline Assessment.* Brighton: Sussex Cancer Network (a local audit published in February 2010), http://info.cancerresearchuk.org/prod_consump/groups/cr_common/@nre/@hea/documents/generalcontent/013995.pdf

Scan the relevant information on bowel cancer prevention and detection in the two documents, keeping the above research statement in mind.

Based on Student Examples 7.1 and 7.2, in no more than 100 words summarize your analysis of these two pieces of grey literature. Discuss your findings with another student or bring these to your next action learning set meeting.

To summarize, we have suggested one way of presenting the research findings from your comprehensive literature review, which is to divide the literature you have reviewed and analyzed into the three distinct groups. We have also demonstrated how you could describe your findings from these three groups in terms of the relevant research questions/statements. By presenting your findings in this way, you have paved the way for the next research process, which will include critical discussion and providing a clear audit trail of how your categories and themes have arisen.

7.3 Discuss the findings by focusing on one theme at a time

This stage of the research process is the most important, yet the most time-consuming part of your comprehensive literature review. You need to demonstrate the process of thematic development by discussing how the data were analyzed and synthesized. To give it justice, the structure of this section of your comprehensive literature review must be carefully considered. We would suggest that you structure your discussion in separate chapters, each related to one of the overarching themes that have arisen from your analysis and synthesis. This is in tune with the pluralistic stance of the mixed methodology of the comprehensive literature review. Within each chapter, you must deliberate on the methodological rigour of each piece of literature reviewed, and how your findings compare with other research and/or existing theories. The use of triangulation and a clear audit trail are also important considerations in boosting the rigour of your comprehensive literature review. Finally, one very important point to remember here is that the three ethical principles of integrity, transparency and accountability must be kept constantly in mind by the researcher when considering rigour (see Chapter 3). Figure 7.1 illustrates the interrelationship of these concepts.

In the following sections, each of the four ways of boosting rigour (as illustrated in Figure 7.1) will be discussed separately.

7.3.1 Methodological rigour or quality of each piece of literature

Rigour is a term that alludes to quality in research and is a subjective phenomenon. The application of a set of objectively determined criteria to measure quality

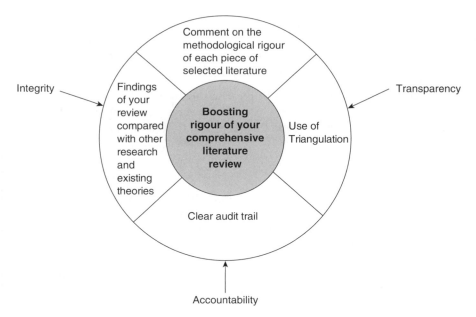

Figure 7.1   Boosting rigour of your comprehensive literature review

goes against the principle of judging quality itself, particularly in qualitative research (Rolfe, 2006; Akkerman et al., 2008; Barusch et al., 2011). However, as a novice researcher, you need to start somewhere. In Chapters 3 and 5, we mentioned the use of the three ethical concepts of integrity, transparency and accountability to guide a generic assessment of the literature. Following on from there, the specific findings from your evaluative criteria (summarized in your data extraction tables) can be used to discuss the rigour or quality of the methodology employed in each paper.

We cannot over-emphasize the importance of determining the quality of each piece of literature in relation to its methodological rigour, as empirical researchers endeavour to maintain data convergence (Sandelowski et al., 2007). This is probably one of the most vital criteria that differentiate the comprehensive literature review methodology from any other type of literature review. At the end of the day, a good quality research project is judged not solely on the merits of its findings, but also on the process by which the researchers arrived at the findings themselves. This requires methodological rigour.

With any piece of empirical research, there are both strengths and weaknesses in its methodological processes. This spans the initial stage of developing the research question/statement to the final stage of reporting of findings. Your judgement of what is of merit in a piece of literature must be justified, along with the flaws that you have identified. Student Example 7.3 demonstrates how this is done.

Student Example 7.3   Discussing methodological merits and flaws of literature related to a specific theme

This example relates to the research on 'The role of the midwife in establishing relationships with clients'. Various types of literature were analyzed and several themes were created. One of these themes is used to illustrate how methodologies can be discussed.

The value of midwife-led care

The value of midwife-led care contributes to the bond between midwife and women and birth partners. Midwives' involvement with the women and their families during the antenatal, intrapartum and postnatal periods provides a continuation of care which has been demonstrated by numerous research reports to enhance the women's childbirth outcomes and experiences.

Overall, the findings indicated that both women and birth partners were satisfied with the care they received from midwife-led services or

---

midwifery group practices. The randomized controlled trial by Harvey et al. (2002) and the postal survey by Symon et al. (2011) both compared midwife-led versus doctor-led units. Samples were sufficiently large to reflect consensus (Punch, 2003). Although these two pieces of research were carried out in different parts of the world, their findings were unanimously in favour of midwife-led services. Harvey et al.'s study tended to be dated as changes would have occurred in healthcare systems in Canada in the last decade.

Fereday et al.'s Australian study (2009) utilized a mixed methodology. Qualitative findings were obtained by using open-ended questions from a self-developed Maternity Satisfaction Questionnaire, which was sent to 84 women enrolled in a continuous midwifery care model. They identified themes such as continuity of care, accessibility and positive attributes of the midwife. These findings reinforced the structured part of the questionnaire, which showed positive scoring on all questions relating to satisfaction with the midwifery care model. This piece of research highlights the strength of mixed methodology as the findings from both quantitative and qualitative parts of the questionnaire were triangulated (Teddlie and Tashakorri, 2009).

The two most recent studies collected data from birth partners. Symon et al. (2011) and Hildingsson et al. (2011) both utilized survey questionnaires sent to over 500 birth partners respectively. The respondents from Symon et al.'s UK study rated birth surroundings and midwifery care as better than the doctor-led units, whereas respondents in Hildingsson et al.'s Swedish study were more specific with their reporting, as the fathers highlighted midwifery support, midwife's presence and information-giving as important aspects of their positive experience.

We have shown you a brief example of how the quality of four papers (three quantitative research studies and one using mixed methodology) were analyzed and reported. We stress the importance of *commenting on both merits and flaws of the methodologies* of this empirical research. In this example, the judgements we have made on the quality of these research studies were justified by referring to research theories by Punch (2003) and Teddlie and Tashakorri (2009).

The findings from these four pieces of literature were discussed under one heading, which was *theme-based*. The purpose of this was to allow the reader to follow the process of thematic development.

The next two sections introduce you to *triangulation* and *audit trail* as means of boosting rigour in your research. These are important concepts as the quality of empirical studies is measured by how well researchers achieve these. Equally important in the comprehensive literature review methodology, you need to demonstrate that these concepts are considered in the process of analysis and synthesis of findings from the literature.

7.3.2 Use of triangulation to boost rigour

Triangulation is a concept whereby a researcher has taken a multiple perspective on a subject under study (Flick, 2009). In the 1970s Denzin and Lincoln developed the concept of triangulation for social research and described four types of triangulation (Denzin and Lincoln, 2005):

- Data or data source triangulation – collecting data from multiple sources, such as from different dates, times and persons
- Investigator triangulation – using more than one researcher to collect and analyze data
- Theory triangulation – using a combination of quantitative and qualitative paradigms to approach data from multiple perspectives
- Methodological triangulation – using several data collecting methods.

Casey and Murphy (2009) examine the role of triangulation in nursing research. They claim that triangulation describes the combination of quantitative and qualitative research, providing a more holistic account of the phenomenon under study. Silverman (2010) advocates that triangulation needs to be carefully thought through by researchers as the concept needs to be in tune with the rest of the research design.

Of the four versions of triangulation mentioned above, there are two that are of particular value in the comprehensive literature review methodology:

1 **Theory triangulation** – The findings from both empirical and non-empirical literature are cross-validated in order to arrive at a theme that is a composite of perspectives (as discussed in Chapter 6). This helps to confirm data convergence (Sandelowski et al., 2007), which in turn promotes quality in this type of research.
2 **Data source triangulation** – Here, different sources of literature are assessed, such as research-based literature as well as government policy documents.

Investigator and methodological triangulation may not be appropriate for you as a student researcher when you are the sole investigator. However, in team research, these two types of triangulation can play an important part in boosting rigour. Team research can promote inter-observer or inter-rater reliability (Parahoo, 2006; Polit and Beck, 2010) in all stages of the literature review research process. Members of the research team can share the task of searching for literature, comparing findings from literature appraisal right through to the synthesis of themes as mentioned in Paterson et al. (2001). Student Example 7.4 illustrates the use of theory and data source triangulation.

Student Example 7.4   Triangulation of findings from literature related to a specific theme

Here we are using the same example of the research on 'The role of the midwife in establishing relationships with clients'. Various pieces of literature were analyzed and several themes were created. One of these themes is used to illustrate how the findings from literature are triangulated and discussed.

Communication between midwife and client

Communication as a two-way process in midwifery care is vital as it helps to establish trust and confidence in the whole process of childbirth. Communication is not just about how the information is delivered, but also about what is being relayed. There is an increase in women seeking information from sources other than healthcare professionals. Midwives need to be cognisant of this fact and be aware of directing women to and providing them with the right information.

Two empirical studies carried out in the UK were analyzed. These looked at communication between midwives and women at antenatal clinics. They were dated from 2006 to 2010. The findings from these research studies were examined alongside that of Standard 22 on 'Communication' in the government report titled *Standards for Maternity Care: Report of a Working Party*, published in June 2008 by the Royal College of Obstetricians and Gynaecologists (RCOG).

The study by McCourt (2006), conducted in the UK, indicated that conventional midwifery care was less conducive to good communication than the newly introduced case-load model of midwifery care. Of the 40 analyzed observations and interviews, it was found that the case-load model utilized a less hierarchical and more conversational form of communication, which offered women greater information, choice and control. The aspect of choice and time to reflect on information given was also highlighted in Standard 22.5 of the maternity care report (RCOG, 2008). The main weakness of the research by McCourt was bias created by the presence of the researcher at the antenatal visits in the form of the 'Hawthorne effect' (Holden, 2001; Parahoo, 2006), which may have impacted on the performance of the midwives and the reactions of the women at the antenatal clinics.

In the second UK research study, conducted by Raine et al. (2010), qualitative methods were again used to collect data in the form of focus groups and semi-structured interviews. The communication experiences of 30 pregnant women were explored. Results showed a variation of good and bad communication. Styles of communication featured prominently with positive comments such as empathetic conversational style and openness to questions. Standard 22.1 of the maternity care report (RCOG, 2008) emphasized the need for training for healthcare professionals so that information can be communicated in an effective and sensitive manner. The use of effective systems of communication was also suggested in Standard 22.2 of the maternity care report (RCOG, 2008). This was picked up on in Raine et al.'s research (2010) where health providers were using text messaging as a means of antenatal clinic appointment reminders, which was seen as constructive by women. All in all, Standard 22 on 'Communication' in the maternity care report (RCOG, 2008) gave health professionals clear guidelines for high-quality care and self-audit. However, the standard setting process was based on 50 source documents, which tended to be previous government reports and reports from organizations with interests in childbirth. There needs to be more unbiased evidence-based information available for both providers and users of maternity services. This is one area that is lacking in this report.

The above example illustrates the use of *theory triangulation* by comparing and contrasting the findings from two qualitative research studies with that of a report on maternity care in the UK. This is the start of the process of data convergence as categories such as 'communication styles' and 'information choices' were beginning to emerge from the literature. The process of interpretation from findings needs to be made transparent.

Data were obtained from both empirical and non-empirical sources (*data source triangulation*). The findings from these, in the form of categories and themes, were cross-validated with each other, which in turn strengthens the process of theme development.

Critique of methodological rigour was offered on both McCourt's (2006) study and the maternity care report (RCOG, 2008). This is an important element in the 'Discussion' chapter of a research project, which helps to boost rigour.

7.3.3 The need to demonstrate an audit trail

Auditing is a term used in business and accounting whereby the auditor or accountant checks over the accounts of a business. This process of auditing eliminates the possibility of error or fraud in fiscal terms. Just as the auditor examines the ledger and provides a detailed account of how money is accrued and spent, the researcher needs to provide a detailed picture or an audit trail of the various research processes. This entails explicit discussion of the decisions taken about the theoretical, methodological and analytical choices throughout the study and the rationale for these decisions (Koch, 2006).

In other words, an audit trail is a record of the steps taken throughout the whole research process. Anfara et al. (2002) (in Barusch et al., 2011) claim that this requires not only good record keeping, but also accountability and transparency on the part of the researcher. Again, this refers to the ethical principles mentioned in Chapters 3 and 5. In adopting the comprehensive literature review methodology, you, as a researcher, need to be aware of and be true to the ethics of research. An honest reflective account of each stage of your research process will provide a record of the decisions you have made and the judgement you have shown along the way, and will subsequently help illuminate the whole process. Student Activity 7.2 is a suggested checklist you can use.

STUDENT ACTIVITY 7.2

Take into account the following questions when auditing your research:

Identifying the research problem/topic

- What is the origin of your research problem/topic?
- Have you discussed your research problem/topic with your supervisor?

Deciding on the right research methodology

- How have you arrived at the decision to use the comprehensive literature review methodology?
- What other research approaches have you considered?

Choosing the sample, sampling process and data collection methods

- What made you decide on the type of literature for your research?
- How did you access the literature?
- What criteria did you use to decide which literature to include/exclude? Why?

Considering ethics when critiquing

- What efforts did you make to follow the ethical principles of integrity, transparency and accountability when critiquing the selected literature?
- What are your rationales for using the chosen critique framework(s) to construct your data extraction tool?

Analyzing data and development of themes

- What theoretical underpinning and processes did you follow when analyzing and synthesizing your data?
- What are the steps you followed in the formation of categories and themes?

Discussing findings with recommendations for practice

- What methods have you used to ensure rigour in your research?
- How significant are your findings in providing recommendations for change?

In our experience in guiding undergraduate and postgraduate students in writing up their comprehensive literature review research projects, we have advocated an end-of-chapter reflective discussion of what, how and why certain aspects of the research 'journey' have impacted on the whole research process. This record of the students' decision processes has provided vital clues to the justification of their audit trail.

7.3.4 Compare your findings with your initial literature review and/or existing theories

The man of science has learnt to believe in justification, not by faith, but by verification.

(Thomas Huxley, English biologist 1825–1895)

This is another important aspect of your discussion because to justify your action or decision is to demonstrate your understanding of a proposition or belief. It is therefore essential not just to state what you have found, but also to support your findings with other reliable sources, such as:

- Findings from research that you have encountered in your initial literature review
- Theories on research methods and methodology – it is important to insert these in your discussion so as to substantiate a point made in relation to the quality of a piece of research
- Other theories, e.g. those in nursing and social psychology are also useful in the defence of your argument (see Student Example 7.5).

Student Example 7.5   The use of other research and theories to justify the discussion of findings

Remember the research on public versus healthcare professionals' viewpoints on the prevention and detection of bowel cancer mentioned earlier on in this chapter. In this example, we have chosen one theme to illustrate the importance of comparing your findings with other research and existing theories.

The emphasis of detection in the expense of prevention of bowel cancer

According to UK cancer statistics based on data collected in 2008–2009 by the Office for National Statistics, bowel cancer is the third most common cancer in the UK after breast cancer and lung cancer. Although the incidence and prevalence of this type of cancer varies with age, gender and genetic inheritance, there is also considerable research evidence to indicate that bowel cancer can be prevented by lifestyle changes (Cancer Research UK, 2011). These findings are reinforced by recently published meta-analysis of prospective studies by Parkin (2011a, 2011b) and Parkin and Boyd (2011a, 2011b and 2011c) in the *British Journal of Cancer*. Their findings identified the role of meat and fibre intake and physical exercise as causative factors in bowel cancer.

Research on screening for bowel cancer has shown that early detection decreases mortality rates in developed countries by as much as 30% and the

---

benefits of national and international bowel cancer screening programmes are irrefutable (Center et al., 2009). Goodyear et al. (2008) highlighted that the increase in public awareness through the UK bowel cancer screening project in the West Midlands had positive impacts, such as reduced emergency admissions, treatment and mortality rates from bowel cancer. However, the national uptake of this screening programme involving faecal occult blood testing had been low (Chapple et al., 2008; von Wagner et al., 2009).

The cost of secondary prevention (FOB testing and flexible signmoidoscopies) is far in excess of primary prevention through education of the public. UK policy makers are in favour of secondary prevention as changing public attitudes towards the prevention of bowel cancer can take time. This may be explained by the attitude change theory cited by McQuire (1985) in Smith and Mackie (2007). There are internal influences on attitude change, such as persistent persuasive messaging from significant others; this is particularly the case when change in attitude impacts on health-related behaviour. Simon et al. (2011) interviewed healthcare professionals who believed that information about cancer should focus on improvements achieved through preventing and treating cancer. This was reinforced by findings from Chapple et al.'s research conducted in 2008. However, in the present socio-economic climate, the public is less likely to consider lifestyle changes in the form of modification of diet and increase in exercise. There is a need, therefore, for external influences to change the public's attitude to cancer prevention, such as social change. For example, food regulation policies and public advertising by the government should be further explored.

The above example has illustrated that *research included in your initial literature review* can be incorporated in your discussion of findings to further illuminate a point, such as the ones mentioned above by Parkin and Boyd (2011a, 2011b, and 2011c), Parkin (2011a, 2011b) and Simon et al. (2011). Equally importantly, *traditional theories*, such as the attitude change theory, can be utilized to explain and justify your findings.

However, it is worthwhile to note that we have not discussed the methodological rigour of any of the pieces of empirical evidence quoted. This is because the above example is fictitious. We advise that you use the analysis of methodological rigour to support the discussion of findings in the above example.

7.4 Strengths and limitations of your comprehensive literature review

The final chapter in your discussion of findings includes two important sections:

1 The strengths and limitations of your research.
2 Recommendations for practice, education and further research.

These sections can be written as a separate chapter, rather than being tagged on to the end of the 'presentation and discussion of findings' chapter. They act as a summary of your comprehensive literature review. We suggest that you refer back to Student Activity 7.2 in this chapter, as the answers you have provided in auditing the stages of your research will come in useful here. The reflective accounts that you have written along the way detail significant aspects of your journey in doing and writing up this research project. You need to be reflexive and be able to stand back from the research and look at it with fresh eyes. Being up close to the project may result in myopic interpretations. In some cases, talking it through with someone not involved in your studies may help you open up further avenues of thought.

7.4.1 Highlight the strengths and be truthful about the limitations

It is just as vital to highlight what has gone right with your research project as it is to focus on the limitations. Being able to examine both strengths and limitations in a balanced manner demonstrates your ability to be insightful and realistic – the essence of reflexivity.

The strength of your research in relation to the appropriateness of research design can be mentioned again here, but be mindful not to repeat what you have said in the methodology chapter. The efforts you have made to ensure methodological rigour in order to arrive at the findings can also be summarized. On personal and professional development, you may wish to indicate the way in which this research has honed your research skills, your ability to evaluate evidence and base your clinical decisions on trustworthy evidence.

It is important to be honest when commenting on the limitations of your comprehensive literature review. Owning up to limitations and explaining how you have attempted to resolve these in your comprehensive literature review are key considerations in this last stage of the research process. The following are some questions to help you identify the limitations:

- What skills and experience that are lacking (in you as the researcher) might have impacted on the quality of your research?
- What problems did you encounter in choosing the sample literature? How did you deal with these?
- How suitable were the chosen frameworks for constructing your data extraction tool and its utilization for analysis?
- How did you overcome problems (if any) with analyzing and synthesizing the data?
- In what ways are your findings related to your own philosophical underpinnings?
- To what extent are your findings specific to a particular socio-cultural context (thereby limiting their generalizability)?
- Are there threats to the rigour or quality of the research?

It is your ability to define these limitations and detail how you went about resolving them that makes a piece of research successful and elevates it above others.

7.4.2 The implications of your findings for practice, education and further research

Finally, you have arrived at the exciting part of your research – when you contemplate the implications of your research findings and make recommendations for change. Research is about solving a problem or illuminating a topic (as mentioned in Chapter 1). Your findings are important as they have the potential to yield new insight and add to a body of knowledge on a topic. This can then instigate change in nursing and midwifery practice and enhance client care.

To help you think of these recommendations, we would suggest the use of the SMART acronym devised by Doran (1981). It was designed initially for strategic planning in management, particularly in the area of goal setting. However, it can be adapted for use here:

- 'S' for specific

The recommendations you make need to contribute to your profession. Think of how these findings can impact on professional practice and the way in which nurses and midwives are educated. Further research may be needed to continue with the investigation of your research topic.

- 'M' for measurable

The recommendations you make depend on how far the findings of your research can be generalized to other settings. It is important to take this into account, as your findings may well reach a wider audience.

- 'A' for achievable

The recommendations you make must be achievable and realistic and reflect the complexity of the current practice environment. These complexities can present barriers to the implementation of research findings, particularly when resources are scarce.

- 'R' for relevant

The recommendations you make need to be relevant to the persons who read them. This boils down to how the research findings are disseminated. Although you are doing this research project as part of your degree studies, there is also an ethical obligation to ensure that the findings of your research are disseminated. You may plan to have a presentation within your student group or publication in the university or hospital magazine. Whatever medium you use, it is important to think of these recommendations and how relevant they are to others.

- 'T' for time-related

The recommendations you make need to be relevant to current nursing and midwifery practice. You may be looking at a topic that is dated. In this case, your recommendations need to suggest ways of applying your findings to what is current at this moment in time.

The above SMART model is aimed at getting you to think through ways to promote your findings in the form of recommendations that practitioners can find useful in practice. Dogherty et al. (2010) have shown that evidence-based practice is spurious and the utilization of research in practice needs to be facilitated. Gerrish et al. (2011) looked at the use of clinical leaders as one of the ways of promoting evidence-based practice among front-line nurses (and midwives). Another is the involvement of students by developing their research appraisal skills and working with research project teams in implementing findings in practice (Putnam and Riggs, 2010). These pieces of research have demonstrated the importance of using research findings in a proactive way to improve nursing and midwifery practice. Finally, Student Activity 7.3 will help you think through your research findings in order to produce useful recommendations.

▬▬▬▬▬ STUDENT ACTIVITY 7.3 ▬▬▬▬▬

List the findings from your comprehensive literature review by reading and re-reading your 'findings' chapters. Your findings are focused on the overarching themes arising from your analysis and synthesis.

Think of the recommendations you could make for the following three areas:

1 For practice
2 For education
3 For further research

Use the SMART framework as a checklist to ensure that the implications for change are considered.

Discuss your findings with your supervisor and bring these to your next action learning set meeting.

End-of-Chapter Learning Points

We hope you have had time to reflect on what you have learnt from the student activities. The following are some of the key points highlighted in this chapter:

1 The essence of presenting and discussing your findings is to get across to your research supervisor and others who read your research report that the findings are arrived at rigorously and succinctly.
2 There are several ways of ensuring methodological rigour and these need to be considered in every chapter when you are discussing the findings.
3 The three ethical principles of integrity, transparency and accountability must be in the forefront of your mind when considering rigour and in discussing the findings of your research.
4 A balanced portrayal of the strengths and limitations of your comprehensive literature review is part and parcel of ensuring reflexivity as a researcher.
5 Your recommendations for change are your 'final words', but they are the most significant words in your research. They must therefore be carefully considered and written in a manner that resounds with the profession. (N.B. Your recommendations *must* be based on what you have found in your comprehensive literature review.)

References

On bowel cancer

Cancer Research UK (2011) Bower cancer statistics. [online] Available at: http://info. cancerresearchuk.org/cancerstats/types/bowel/incidence/uk-bowel-cancer-incidence-statistics [Accessed 13 February 2012].

Center, M.M., Jemal, A., Smith, R.A. and Ward E. (2009) 'Worldwide variations in colorectal cancer', *CA: A Cancer Journal for Clinicians*, 59(6), 366–378.

Chapple, A., Ziebland, S., Hewitson, P. and McPherson, A. (2008) 'What affects the uptake of screening for bowel cancer using a faecal occult blood test (FOBt): a qualitative study', *Social Science & Medicine*, 66(12), 2425–2435.

Goodyear, S.J., Leung, E., Menon, A., Pedamallu, S., William, N. and Wong, L.S. (2008) 'The effects of population-based faecal occult blood test screening upon emergency colorectal cancer admissions in Coventry and north Warwickshire', *Gut*, 57, 218–222.

McQuire, W.J. (1985) 'Attitude and attitude change' cited in G. Lindzey and E. Aronson (eds) (1985) *Handbook of Social Psychology* (3rd edn). New York: Random House.

Parkin, D.M. (2011a) '5. Cancers attributable to dietary factors in the UK in 2010 – meat consumption', *British Journal of Cancer*, 105, S24–S26.

Parkin, D.M. (2011b) '9. Cancers attributable to inadequate physical exercise in the UK in 2010', *British Journal of Cancer*, 105, S38–S41.

Parkin, D.M. and Boyd, L. (2011a) '4. Cancers attributable to dietary factors in the UK in 2010 – low consumption of fruit and vegetables', *British Journal of Cancer*, 105, S19–S23.

Parkin, D.M. and Boyd, L. (2011b) '6. Cancers attributable to dietary factors in the UK in 2010 – low consumption of fibre', *British Journal of Cancer*, 105, S27–S30.

Parkin, D.M. and Boyd, L. (2011c) '8. Cancers attributable to overweight and obesity in the UK in 2010', *British Journal of Cancer*, 105, S34–S37.

Simon, A.E., Wardle, J. and Miles, A. (2011) 'Is it time to change the stereotype of cancer: the expert view?', *Cancer Causes Control*, 22, 135–140.

Smith, E.R. and Mackie, D.M. (2007) *Social Psychology* (3rd edn). Philadelphia, PA: Psychology Press.

von Wagner, C., Good, A., Wright, D., Rachet, B., Obichere, A., Bloom, S. and Wardle, J. (2009) 'Inequalities in colorectal cancer screening participation in the first round of the national screening programme in England', *British Journal of Cancer*, 101, S60–S63.

On midwifery care

Fereday, J., Collins, C., Turnbull, D. and Pincombe, J. (2009) 'An evaluation of midwifery group practice. Part II: women's satisfaction', *Women and Birth*, 22(1), 11–16.

Harvey, S., Rach, D., Stainton, M.C., Jarrell, J. and Brant, R. (2002) 'Evaluation of satisfaction with midwifery care', *Midwifery*, 18(4), 260–267.

Hildingsson, I., Cederlof, L. and Widên, S. (2011) 'Fathers' birth experience in relation to midwifery care', *Women and Birth*, 24(3), 129–136.

McCourt, C. (2006) 'Supporting choice and control? Communication and interaction between midwives and women at the antenatal booking visit', *Social Science and Medicine*, 62(6), 1307–1318.

Raine, R., Cartwright, M., Richens, Y., Mahamed, Z. and Smith, D. (2010) 'A qualitative study of women's experiences of communication in antenatal care: identifying areas for action', *Maternal and Child Health Journal*, 14(4), 590–599.

Royal College of Obstetricians and Gynaecologists with Royal College of Midwives (2008) *Standards for Maternity Care: Report of a Working Party*. London: RCOG Press. Available at: www.rcog.org.uk/files/rcog-corp/uploaded-files/WPRMaternityStandards2008.pdf.

Symon, A.G., Dugard, P., Butchart, M., Carr, V. and Paul, J. (2011) 'Care and environment in midwife-led and obstetric-led units: a comparison of mothers' and birth partners' perceptions', *Midwifery*, 27(6), 880–886.

On research and rigour

Akkerman, S., Admiraal, W., Brekelmans, M. and Oost, H. (2008) 'Auditing quality of research in social sciences', *Quality and Quantitiy*, 42(2), 257–274.

Anfara, Jr. V.A., Brown, K.M. and Mangione, T.L. (2002) Qualitative analysis on stage: making the research process more public, *Educational Researcher*, 31, 28 – 38. Available at: www.edr.sagepub.com/cgi/content/abstract/31/7/28 (accessed 25 September 2012)

Barusch, A., Gringeri, C. and George, M. (2011) 'Rigor in qualitative social work research: a review of strategies used in published articles', *Social Work Research*, 35(1), 11–19.

Casey, D. and Murphy, K. (2009) 'Issues in using methodological triangulation in research', *Nurse Researcher*, 16(4), 40–55.

Denzin, N.K. and Lincoln, Y.S. (eds) (2000) *Handbook of Qualitative Research* (2nd edn). London: Sage.

Doran, G.T. (1981) 'There's a S.M.A.R.T. way to write management goals and objectives', *Management Review*, 70(11), 35–36.

Flick, U. (2009) *An Introduction to Qualitative Research*. London: Sage.

Holden, J.D. (2001) 'Hawthorne effects and research into professional practice', *Journal of Evaluation in Clinical Practice*, 7(1), 65–70.

Koch, T. (2006) 'Establishing rigour in qualitative research: a decision trail', *Journal of Advanced Nursing*, 53(1), 91–103.

Parahoo, K. (2006) *Nursing Research: Principles, Process and Issues* (2nd edn). Basingstoke: Palgrave Macmillan.

Paterson, B.L., Thorne, E.S., Cannan, C. and Jillings, C. (2001) *Meta-Study of Qualitative Health Research: A Practical Guide to Meta-Analysis and Meta-Synthesis*. Thousand Oaks, CA: Sage.

Polit, D.F. and Beck, C.T. (2010) *Essentials of Nursing Research: Appraising Evidence for Nursing Practice* (7th edn). Philadelphia, PA: Wolters Kluwer Health/Lippincott Williams and Wilkins.

Punch, K.F. (2003) *Survey Research: The Basics*. London: Sage.

Rolfe, G. (2006) 'Validity, trustworthiness and rigour: quality and the idea of qualitative research', *Journal of Advanced Nursing*, 53(3), 304–310.

Sandelowski, M., Barroso, J. and Voils, I.C. (2007) 'Using qualitative metasummary to synthesize qualitative and quantitative descriptive findings', *Research in Nursing and Health*, 30(1), 99–111.

Silverman, D. (2010) *Doing Qualitative Research* (3rd edn). London: Sage.

Teddlie, C.B. and Tashakorri, A. (2009) *Foundations of Mixed Methods Research: Integrating Quantitative and Qualitative Approaches in the Social and Behavioural Sciences*. London: Sage.

On evidence-based practice

Dogherty, E., Harrison, M. and Graham, I. (2010) 'Facilitation as a role and process in achieving evidence-based practice in nursing: a focused review of concept and meaning', *Worldview on Evidence-based Nursing, Sigma Theta Tau International Honor Society of Nursing*, 7(2), 76–89.

Gerrish, K., Guillaume, L., Kirshbaum, M., McDonnell, A. and Nolan, M. (2011) 'Factors influencing the contribution of advanced practice nurses to promote evidence-based practice among front-line nurses: findings from a cross-sectional survey', *Journal of Advanced Nursing*, 67(5), 1079–1090.

Putnam, J.M. and Riggs, C.J. (2010) 'Involving students in the real world of evidence-based practice', *Journal of Nursing Education*, 49(7), 423–424.

EIGHT

Writing Your Research Report

┌─── **Aim and objectives** ───┐

The aim of this chapter is to provide realistic and practical ideas in writing up your research project. By the end of the chapter you will be able to:

- Structure your research project by considering the following:
  - layout
  - language and writing style
  - other formal issues
- Adhere to the process of writing up by taking note of:
  - the time allocation
  - intellectual, physical and psychosocial support mechanisms
- Be aware of the outcome of your research by:
  - revisiting the initial aim and objectives of your research project
  - questioning yourself and reflecting on a number of important issues.

8.1 Introduction

A research project is an extended piece of work that demonstrates your ability to search, research and write independently on a topic of your choice. It is sometimes called a project[1] or a thesis (the name varies between universities and may depend on the level of study). Undergraduate and postgraduate courses prefer the term 'dissertation', whereas doctoral studies culminate in a thesis. For this chapter, we will be using the term 'research project'.

Your research project is the final piece of course work which contributes to your degree classification. In most universities, this frequently amounts to double or triple (sometimes quadruple) the weighting of a normal assignment. Although there is a certain amount of variability between universities and within faculties of one university, you can calculate how much your project is worth by looking at the credit weighting of your research dissertation module. This credit weighting is part of the Credit Accumulation and Transfer Scheme (CATS) that allows students to move between courses within one university or between universities.

This research project means a lot to students because it reflects the amount of effort you have put into this piece of work and to the course generally. The process itself is invaluable as it develops you as a researcher by providing you with problem-solving and higher-order intellectual skills. The grade awarded to research projects carries other connotations to different people, such as pro-spective employers. It is not uncommon for employers to ask to see research projects and/or pose questions related to applicants' research at interviews. When jobs are scarce, employers need to use other means to gauge applicants' abilities.

Each university has its own guidelines for students on how to write and pre-sent their research projects. These guidelines also provide the criteria for judg-ing the quality of these projects. The government has a quality assurance body that oversees the standard of teaching and assessment across a whole range of courses. They are particularly concerned with the transparency of marking crite-ria for research projects and their interpretation by both students and teachers (Quality Assurance Agency, 2006). It is therefore important for students to be prepared, as there is so much to be done and discover before you embark on your final-year write-up. Getting to grips with the marking criteria is only one of the things to bear in mind when writing up your research project. The rest of this chapter will provide you with practical advice by looking at the structure, process and outcome of your research project.

8.2 The structure of your research project

In the majority of universities, courses are designed to incorporate a research module early on in the second year, whereby students are encouraged to start thinking about the topic of their research project. You may be asked to conduct a preliminary literature review and to write up a research proposal, which is submit-ted as an end-of-module assessment. This is an invaluable exercise as the proposal not only makes you focus on a topic for your research, but will motivate you to think of the structure of the project to come.

As part of the research proposal, you may have to submit a timetable or a Gantt chart.[2] Figure 8.1 is an example of a research timetable/chart based on a six-month period.

	Months of the research project					
	1	**2**	**3**	**4**	**5**	**6**
1. Form a research project support group						
2. Conduct a preliminary literature review						
3. Decide on your research topic/problem						
3. Refine your research topic with your supervisor						
4. Compose a timetable for completion						
5. Read other research projects in library						
6. Adjust and refine your methodology						
7. Schedule data collection and begin collecting						
8. Read and re-read the literature						
9. Analyze and synthesize the literature						
10. Interpret the findings						
11. Synthesize findings into themes						
12. Revise the proposal into research report format						
13. Write your research report						
14. Submit the research report draft to your supervisor						
15. Completed in its final version of your research report						
16. Take research report for printing or prepare to submit online						
17. Submit the research report						

Figure 8.1   Research project timetable

The research project module in most universities is launched at the beginning of your final year at university. You will be given a module handbook and it is important that you examine this handbook closely for the following:

1 A suggested layout for the presentation of the project in the various chapter headings (see section 8.2.3 for an example).
2 The assessment criteria for the marking of the project (see section 8.2.4.1).
3 The word limit and the final submission date (see section 8.2.4.2).

There will be other details in the handbook that may vary between different faculties and/or universities. It is good practice for you to go through these and discuss any queries with the module leader and/or your research supervisor.

It is also good practice to look at other research projects written by past students. There is always a selection of these in hard copy or DVD format available for students to review in the reference sections of libraries. Avoid looking at past research projects that are only awarded high grades as it is just as useful to examine those which are awarded lower grades (where these are available). You can then compare the different qualities of these pieces of submitted work. There is also a lot to learn from looking at research projects produced by students from other faculties to compare the way in which research was conducted. If you do not have the opportunity to look at other students' research projects before you start your project, it is never too late to look at them afterwards as they will give you ideas as to how you should write up your work.

8.2.1 Layout of the project

Once you have arrived at the stage of writing up your research project, you will feel a great sense of achievement... and so you should – well done! The next and final step is to write up what you have done. It is important that you focus on the layout of your research project as you want to present your work in such a way that it reflects the degree of effort you have put in to solving the research problem or to illuminating the topic you have investigated. Student Activity 8.1 will help you focus on the layout of your research project.

STUDENT ACTIVITY 8.1

Study your research project module handbook and make a list of the suggested layout points. Then make a couple more lists of the same information from previous students' research projects you have read in the library.

(Continued)

(Continued)

Compare the lists you have made and discuss with another student the similarities and differences. Bring your findings to your next research action learning set or discussion group. It may also be useful to discuss these findings with your research supervisor.

You need to realize that there are no strict rules on how research projects are written and presented. The most important thing to remember is that your research supervisor may well be marking your work, so it is worthwhile to know his/her view on the matter.

8.2.2 Language usage

To present your work in the best possible format, the language you use needs to be in an academic style. The essay-writing skills you have gathered in your years of education will help with this task. However, if you have not been in education for a while and/or you feel out-of-practice in writing academic essays, we would suggest that you consult one of the following books:

Redman, P. (2006) *Good Essay Writing: A Social Sciences Guide* (3rd edn). London: Sage.
Shields, M. (2010) *Essay Writing: A Student's Guide* (Sage Study Skills Series). London: Sage.

One last word before we move on to the next section on writing up the chapters of your research project. There is one query that raises its head with healthcare professional students and that is the use of first and third person in academic writing. There has been a long tradition of using the third person in academic writing and, personally, we would endorse this, but we suggest that you check with your research supervisor as to how he/she feels about its usage. As for the use of first person, it is acceptable to refer to oneself in your writing when you are reflecting on an incident or referring to an account in practice. Student Example 8.1 demonstrates how you can switch from the third to the first person in your writing.

Student Example 8.1   Switching from third person to first person

Speer (2008) reported in a journal article that there is an increase in ophthalmia neonatorum in the USA as a result of sexually transmitted diseases in the mother, in particular that of gonorrhoea and chlamydia. Research evidence gathered from Africa and the USA showed that 22.3% of 452 infants born to HIV-1 infected mothers were diagnosed with neonatal conjunctivitis (Gichuhi et al., 2009), gonorrhoea, chlamydia and staphylococci being the most commonly found pathogens. Both of these reports suggest a need for increased vigilance and prophylaxis for conjunctivitis in these infants. Although the epidemiological evidence in the UK may not echo the situation

---

globally, Pilling et al. (2008) suggested that the under-reporting of cases of conjunctivitis in newborns in England and Wales was due to the failure of clinicians to notify positive cases.

During my community experience with the district midwife in a rural practice, all cases of babies with 'sticky eyes' were followed up closely. There was a strict code of practice that each midwife adhered to, preventative measures being the first line of management, and mothers were given detailed instructions of how to care for their babies' eyes. Eye swabs were always taken and the results relayed back to the mother, and if an organism was identified treatment was given promptly. I personally witnessed the General Practitioner (GP) completing the public health notification, which was sent to the Public Health Epidemiology Department as both a hard copy and as a computerized record.

In the above paragraphs, we have illustrated the interjection of a personal account. This was used as a counter-argument to Pilling et al.'s (2008) findings, which may be out-dated since these authors (although ophthalmologists and epidemiologists) gathered data from case reports between 1997 and 2008. This was before accountability and quality assurance in health care became major concerns for GPs and other care givers.

8.2.3 Writing up the chapters

From Student Activity 8.1 you will have gathered that there are various ways to present your chapters in research projects. The following is one suggestion of how your project can be presented.

Front page or frontispiece (title of research project, full title of your degree, awarding university, your name and year)

Abstract (see section 8.2.3.1)

Acknowledgement (a statement of dedication to individual(s) who had helped you with the process of the research)

Contents page in bullet format (all chapter titles and corresponding page numbers, lists of tables and/or diagrams, references, appendices)

Introduction and the research problem or topic (see section 8.2.3.2)

Methodology chapter on comprehensive literature review (see section 8.2.3.3)

Data collection chapter, including sampling and access to data (see section 8.2.3.4)

Analysis and synthesis chapter, including ethical considerations (see section 8.2.3.5)

Presentation and discussion of findings chapter (see section 8.2.3.6)

Final chapter, including strengths, limitations and recommendations (see section 8.2.3.7)

References in the correct referencing style used by your university

Appendices (referred to sequentially in the chapters and presented in the same order in this last section of the research) (see section 8.2.3.8).

8.2.3.1 How to write the abstract

An abstract is generally viewed as a summary of your research project. However, it is also important to remember that abstracts are the first piece of writing to be read. Therefore, you need to focus on the important aspects of your research findings. It is usually not longer than 300 words and could be presented as a written paragraph or in notations with sub-headings.

The notated version is frequently favoured by healthcare profession students. The following are some suggested headings:

- Aim and research question(s)
- Methodology (sample size and characteristics, analysis techniques)
- Findings
- Conclusions and recommendations

Read your research report several times before you write your abstract. Try not to cut and paste parts of your report into the abstract. It is much better to summarize it in 'new' words, highlighting your findings in an honest but enthusiastic manner.

(One positive note: the word count for your abstract is *not* included in the total word count.)

8.2.3.2 How to write the introduction and the research problem/topic

For a 10,000-word research project, this chapter should be approximately 1,000 words in length (10%). The introduction needs to include the reason(s) for choosing the research topic. The process of identifying the research problem or topic should also be elaborated here. This will include the three important steps advocated in Chapter 2, that is:

- Reflecting on personal experiences
- Seeking colleagues' and clients' perspectives
- Preliminary exploration of literature.

In support of your writing, mind-maps can be included in your appendices. These will illustrate in diagrammatic format the development of your ideas and the evolutionary process of formulating your research problem. This chapter culminates with a set of aim(s) and objectives. If research questions/ statements were formulated, then these should also be included at the end of this chapter.

8.2.3.3 How to write the methodology chapter

This is an important chapter as it demonstrates your understanding of the comprehensive literature review methodology. First, we would like to revisit Crotty's (2003) definition of methodology. He claims that methodology is the strategy, plan of action, process or design lying behind the choice and use of particular methods and linking the choice and use of methods to the desired outcomes. This chapter will require a minimum of 2,000 words out of a 10,000-word research report (20%), as it will include the following:

- Justification of your choice of comprehensive literature review methodology, alongside a clear description of this methodology
- Explanation of the differences between the two contrasting paradigms (quantitative and qualitative) and the need for a pluralist approach in the form of mixed methodology
- Brief discussion of alternative methodologies that you might have considered for this research project.

=== STUDENT ACTIVITY 8.2 ===

From your previous research modules, make brief notes on the pros and cons of the following methodologies.

Quantitative designs

1 Experimental designs (true and quasi-experiments)
2 Surveys

Qualitative designs

3 Phenomenology
4 Grounded theory

Mixed methodologies (see Figure 3.4 in Chapter 3)

5 A mixture of quantitative and qualitative research designs
6 A mixture of two qualitative research designs

Alternative literature review methodology

7 Systematic review

Select from the above list two or three designs and justify why they are *not* suitable for the research topic you have chosen.

This exercise will help to strengthen your argument for using the comprehensive literature review methodology.

8.2.3.4 How to write the data collection chapter

This chapter highlights the decision processes of data selection and collection. In the comprehensive literature review methodology, research findings and grey literature act as secondary sources of data. Your sampling process needs to be clearly articulated in order to demonstrate transparency and to strengthen rigour. A minimum of 1,000 words (out of a 10,000-word research report) is usually required to describe these processes.

Diagrammatic representation in the form of tables will help to summarize your data collection process. As your discussion will be centred on the tables themselves, it is appropriate to keep these in the main text, rather than removing them to the appendices. The areas you will need to focus on in this chapter are as follows:

- The sample and sampling type chosen
- The inclusion and exclusion criteria and your justification
- The searching processes undertaken, such as the search engines you used to help narrow your search (e.g. a table of key words used and the number of hits for each key word)
- The type and range of literature collected (e.g. a table highlighting the final list of empirical and non-empirical literature selected).

8.2.3.5 How to write the analysis and synthesis chapter

This chapter demonstrates your ability to critically analyze and synthesize the selected literature. There are two processes that need to be clearly described and justified:

1. The process of analysis: this will involve the justification of the choice of critique frameworks used and their modification and adaptation for the critique of grey literature. Justification for designing your own critique framework also applies.
2. The process of summarizing the findings from your individual analysis: the use of data extraction or summary tables will be very useful here. These summary tables are normally included in the appendices as they can be very extensive.

A word count of approximately 1,000–2,000 words is required for this chapter (10–20% of a 10,000-word research report).

8.2.3.6 How to write the presentation and discussion of findings

This is the essence of your research report. We suggest 3,000–4,000 words for this chapter (out of a 10,000-word research report). The sections of this chapter will be centred on the themes formulated from your research. In other words, if three themes are formulated, there will be three sections; if four themes, then four sections, and so on. Again, a table will be useful to illustrate the thematic development. Student Example 8.2 illustrates such a table.

Student Example 8.2   Thematic development of two themes in a comprehensive literature review on the 'Role of the midwife in establishing relationships with clients'

Theme One: The value of midwife-led care

The following are the emergent themes and literature that contributed to the development of the above overarching theme:

1   Continuity of care: literature number 3, 9, 10
2   Instilling trust and confidence: literature number 2, 4

Theme Two: Communication between midwife and client

The following are the emergent themes and literature that contributed to the development of the above overarching theme:

1   Communication styles: literature number 1, 2, 3, 5, 6
2   Information choices: literature number 4, 5, 7, 8, 9

From the total of 10 pieces of literature, we have demonstrated how you can display the literature that 'feeds into' the four emergent themes and the two overarching themes.

Depending on how many themes are identified, each theme-based section or chapter in which you discuss the findings from the literature that contributed to this theme will be approximately 1,000 words. There needs to be evidence of critical discussion of the methodological merits and flaws of each piece of literature as well as evidence of triangulation of findings from more than one source (as mentioned in Chapter 7).

8.2.3.7 How to write the final chapter

As with any publication, the last chapter or paragraph often provides the most impact. It is not unusual for markers of research projects to read the final chapter first before reading the rest of the document. This chapter will afford a minimum of 1,000–2,000 words out of a 10,000-word research project. There are vital points to include in this chapter, such as:

- A summary of the findings and recommendations for change in practice
- Identification of the strengths and limitations of your research, and recommendations for future research
- Reflection on some of the significant stages of conducting the research (detailed reflective pieces can be appended), and what you personally have learnt from the process.

8.2.3.8 Appendices

Any information placed at the end of an essay or publication is an appendix or an addendum. These can be in the form of tables, diagrams, pictures or prose. It is unusual to find an appendix of more than 500 words in prose. Appendices should provide information that has a direct relationship to the main body of the essay or publication. We have had students in the past who ran out of words in the main text and decided to place the rest of their written work in the appendix. Unfortunately, these students were misinformed and they failed to pass their assignment because their work was incomplete!

All appendices are numbered or identified alphabetically in the order in which they appear in the main text. Each appendix should be given a title and referred to in the contents page.

STUDENT ACTIVITY 8.3

Select a few research dissertations or projects in the library's reference section and look at their appendices. Make lists of what is in their appendices and examine how the authors have referred to them in the main text, and how they listed them in their contents page.

See if you can find a reflective account in one of the appendices.

Finally, note the differences between how students refer to tables, charts or diagrams in the main text and how they do so in the appendices.

Share your findings with another student or bring them up at your action learning set meetings.

8.2.4 Other formal issues to consider

As the final submission date is looming, you may find it stressful to discover things that you have not considered, such as other 'formal issues'. The following are some examples of these:

- The correct referencing style: most universities advocate the modified Harvard referencing style. As you are referring to a large amount of literature in your research report, we would suggest computer software, such as EndNote, to save you a lot of time and worry. Each university's learning resource department has its own EndNote user manual. We advise you to contact them if you have not already done so.
- The correct font, font size and margin settings: you may have already noted these from writing previous assignments, but there is no harm checking these requirements in your research module handbook.
- Printing and binding of copies of research reports: there is a research report printing and binding service available at each university that is normally free of charge. You need to check the details of this service, such as the provision of hard copies versus temporary storage devices (such as a USB memory stick) for printing. Otherwise, there are on-the-spot printing and binding services at most high street print shops, but they can be costly, especially when several copies are needed.

8.2.4.1 The assessment criteria

The allotment of marks to the research report will be divided according to certain predetermined criteria. It is useful for you to have a clear understanding of what the report is measured against. The following are examples of the areas in which the report is assessed:

- Presentation and use of references
- Understanding of the research topic and research process
- Analysis and synthesis of literature
- Discussion and evaluation of the findings
- Application of findings to practice
- Use of reflection.

Depending on your level of study, the above criteria may vary. The percentage weighting given to each of the above may also differ according to universities or faculties within one university.

STUDENT ACTIVITY 8.4

Although your research module handbook may have provided you with the marking criteria for your research report, you may not have examined it closely. We would suggest that you discuss this with other students at the next action learning set and/or with your research supervisor.

Look at the differences in the marking criteria between Grades A, B, C and D. It is also useful to look at the 'fail' criteria because this is one grade you would want to avoid!

(Continued)

You may also bring up at your action learning set how the marking of research reports are conducted – for example, whether a double-blind marking system is utilized at your school or university for research reports.

You may also want to clarify the role of external examiners, in particular their role in the viva voce examinations (if this applies in your case). A viva voce examination is an additional process set up for some research degrees to assess students. The regulations for the conduct of these are clearly advertised and you need to be familiar with them beforehand. Mock viva voce examinations are essential in ensuring success.

Share your findings with other students as the more you voice your ideas with others, the more you will learn and the wiser you will be.

8.2.4.2 Word limit and submission date

The word limit varies greatly between universities and faculties within one university. Generally, the word limit is as follows:

- undergraduate dissertation or research project: 6,000–10,000 words
- postgraduate dissertation or research project: 8,000–20,000 words

Each double-spaced page of submitted written work contains approximately 250 words. The number of pages for your research project is calculated as follows:

- undergraduate dissertation or research project: 25–40 pages long (excluding references and appendices)
- postgraduate dissertation or research project: 32–80 pages long (excluding references and appendices).

Word limits for research projects need to be adhered to strictly as students are penalized for going over the limit. Again, there are different regulations as to the penalty imposed by universities. It is useful to find out about this beforehand. Recent changes in assessment and examination regulations in universities have brought about a percentage graded penalty system, whereby a percentage of the overall mark is deducted according to the number of words over the limit.

The approximate number of words for each chapter was discussed in section 8.2.3. However, the general rule of thumb for allotting the number of words to the three major sections of your research report cannot be over-emphasized. Both introductory and final chapters should be approximately 10% of the total word count. This leaves approximately 80% of the word count for the main body.

The date for final submission of your research report is another important reference point to keep in mind as this will determine your research timetable. The example of such a timetable/Gantt chart in section 8.2 is based on a six-month period, but it can be adjusted according to the final submission date of your project.

8.3 The process of writing up

A process is a series of actions or changes. As the process of writing up your research project unfolds, you will feel that you have surmounted numerous hurdles to get to this final stage. It is important for you to write up this research in such a way that it achieves the necessary outcome. The series of actions or changes that you have taken or made requires an understanding of your own physical and psycho-social needs. Maslow's hierarchy of needs (Figure 8.2) defines the motivational factors that drive you to achieve your goal (Stephens, 2000).

The following sections will suggest ways in which you can motivate yourself to maximize your potential and achieve the final process of writing up.

8.3.1 A conducive environment (physiological needs)

Space and comfortable surroundings are essential elements in a conducive environment for writing up your research project.

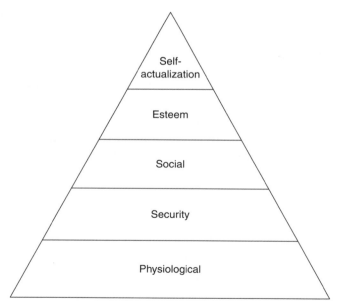

Figure 8.2 Maslow's hierarchy of needs

Think of an ideal environment in which you can place yourself for writing up your research project. Make a list of the essential physical characteristics.

Now, look at the environment you are in at present (it may be student accommodation or similar) and make a similar list.

Try to bridge the two situations and find a compromise. The following is a checklist you can use to help you identify a conducive environment:

✓ Peace and quiet
✓ Warm and cosy
✓ Space for computer and other IT
✓ Close vicinity to amenities (shops, park)

✓ Music, TV and other media
✓ Food and sustenance available
✓ Access to books and journals
✓ Opportunity to meet friends

There may be other demands in your life, such as family responsibilities or commitment to a part-time job. It is therefore also important to take these into account.

Some students may consider spending some time at home with their family, who will provide a better environment for them to think, read and write. Others prefer to stay among friends, who will provide the social and possibly intellectual stimulation needed. We have come across students who have taken refuge in university libraries, as they found solace in solitude and quiet.

8.3.2 Adhering to your timetable (security needs)

In order to feel secure, you need to be in control of the situation you are in. Once your physical environment is sorted out, the next important factor to consider is the time allocation for writing your research project. The Gantt chart in section 8.2 is a month-by-month schedule that you can use to track the progress of your entire research project. The schedule assumes an average 10,000-word research project of 40 pages. This will require approximately a total effort of 500 hours. If this is calculated over a six-month period, then an average of 80–85 hours per month must be devoted to the research project. This assumes that you have no other academic commitments and that the whole six months are available for you to work on your research.

Student Example 8.3   How Anita spent six months on her research project

Anita is a mature student on the nursing degree course. She lives at home with her husband and two school-aged children. Her husband works at home where he has an office.

Prior to the final year of her course, Anita elicited her mother's help to collect the children from school and to help with their homework. Anita's husband took the children to school and Anita collected them from her mother's house when she finished her work-based placement. This worked well for the family, although Anita missed spending more time with her children.

During the six-month research project period, Anita discussed with her husband how best to create a conducive working environment. She made the dining room table her work area, so as not to encroach on her husband's office space. They bought a laptop for Anita to store all her research data and to use the internet. She also renewed her mobile phone contract, so that she could use her new phone to record some of the action learning set discussions and the supervision sessions with her research supervisor.

Anita devised a routine for her day while she was at home for the final writing-up of her project. It was difficult to adhere to it initially as the children were not at school due to holidays. However, she soon caught up with the missed hours and got into a routine of reading in the morning and writing in the afternoon. She took breaks during the day for walks with her husband and they talked about everything other than their work.

From the above scenario, you can see how a student's home and work life have to adapt to the demands of the research project. Share this scenario with others who are significant in your life and see if they can come up with ideas to tackle your physiological and security needs.

8.3.3 Forming a research project support group or action learning sets (social needs)

At this final stage of the research, your social needs play a vital part in ensuring the successful completion of your project. Support groups need to be formed early on in the research project time-line. Most universities facilitate action learning sets for groups of students to meet during this time. These meetings are usually held fortnightly and involve 4–6 students in a group. There is normally a facilitator, who is knowledgeable on research, but not necessarily one of the research project supervisors. In our experience, most students find these meetings helpful as action learning serves a number of purposes:

- Sharing of experiences
- Supporting each other (social, intellectual and emotional support)
- Increasing understanding of research principles and processes
- Transferring what students have learned into their own practice of doing and writing up research projects
- Developing critically reflective and reflexive students, practitioners and academics.

Coghlan and Pedler (2006) advocate action learning as a vital component of successful research projects. The role of the action learning set facilitator is also important in ensuring a clear demarcation of roles within the set, fairness and equity in the ground rules with which the set functions, and open lines of communication between set members and with any other significant individuals whom set members wish to include.

In order to take full advantage of action learning, students should be encouraged to keep reflective logs, which they can either keep private or share with others at their set meetings. As mentioned in Student Example 8.3, individuals can record discussions at set meetings, providing they have the permission of other set members.

8.3.4 Supervisor and student contracts (esteem needs)

Finally, to reach the end goal of completing your research project (i.e. reaching Maslow's state of self-actualization), you need to maintain self-esteem by honouring the contract you have set with your research supervisor. Your supervisor (in the majority of universities) is one of the markers of your research report. In other words, if you have consulted your supervisor and taken heed of the guidance he/she has given you on your research project, then there is a good chance that you may be on the right track! This seems rather simplistic, but you may want to consider the following possible scenarios:

- Students do not always consult their supervisors
- Misunderstandings can occur between student and supervisor regarding the content of discussions at supervisory meetings
- Supervisors are not available or cannot be contacted.

To avoid such happenings, research supervisors are allocated to students early on during their research project period. It is the students' responsibility to contact their supervisor and initiate a meeting. The most important process at this point is for both parties to agree to a supervision contract. The content of a contract may be as follows:

- Number and frequency of supervision meetings
- Process and ways of communicating with each other
- Content of the supervision meetings
- Who else needs to be involved in the supervisory process and on what basis (e.g. a specialist librarian or practice expert may act as a consultant).

The contract between the research supervisor and student is written down and kept in the student's file so that it can be referred to and amended if required. In our experience, this contract helps to set boundaries and prevent misinterpretation (between supervisors and between student and supervisor). Tutorial records can still be written by the supervisor and reflective logs by students, but the research contract is 'sacrosanct'.

8.4 Outcome of your research

You have nearly reached the end. This final goal-post can be crossed if you take note of some vital 'landmarks' during the process of doing your research project.

8.4.1 Keeping a check on your initial aims and objectives

To keep on track, you need to set clear aims and objectives at the onset of your research project. It is therefore useful and important to refer back to your aims and objectives now and again. We have suggested to students in the past that they put their aims and objectives for their research project on a memo-board in their study/work area. This will become a constant reminder. Aims and objectives can be 'movable feasts', but you need to have good justifications to change them, especially if you are over halfway into your research project. We would strongly suggest that you discuss any proposed changes with your research supervisor.

Student Example 8.4   Justification for changing the aims and objectives

Sam is a midwifery student in the final year of her degree course. She has devised a set of aims and objectives for her research project, which were agreed with her supervisor. They are as follows:

The aim of this research project is to conduct a literature review on the use of water births and mothers' experiences using the comprehensive literature review methodology. The following are the objectives:

1 To compare the use of water births nationally and internationally.
2 To examine the information given to mothers and partners on choosing water birth.
3 To understand the effects of water births on both mother and the newborn.
4 To explore mothers' experiences of water births.

(Continued)

She had been working on achieving these until she found several literature sources highlighting partners' experiences of water births. She also discovered that international literature on water births varies greatly in interpretations of what water birth constitutes and how it is facilitated. Sam discussed these issues with her supervisor and between them they decided to focus on the UK perspective, but to include partners' experiences of water birth rather than just focusing on the mothers' experiences.

There are clear justifications for changing the objectives for Sam's research and these were jointly agreed by Sam and her research supervisor.

8.4.2 Questions to ask yourself

Asking questions of yourself is a vital part of the reflective process. In Chapter 1, we suggested some well-known authors who have written about reflection, such as Gibbs (1988), Schön (1991), Johns (2004) etc. They have emphasized retrospective reflection to enable individuals to be prospective thinkers. The following are three key questions you can ask yourself:

- What have you learned from the dissertation or project?
- How has it contributed to your course?
- Why is this important to you?

It is useful to re-examine and reflect on what you have learnt on the course as a whole and how this has contributed to the topic you have chosen for your project. You may have formalized the answers to these questions in your reflections by keeping a log, as mentioned previously. If so, it will be very useful to read over it and use it for material for the last chapter of your research report.

You may also think about the answers to the above questions after the research report has been submitted. They can provide you with key pointers for writing your curriculum vitae or future job applications.

End-of-Chapter Learning Points

We hope you have had time to reflect on what you have learned from the Student Activities. The following are some of the keys points highlighted in this chapter:

1 To write up your research project successfully, you need to be aware of ways to present your work in the most positive light.
2 Structure the project with chapters that are systematic and will make sense to the audience who reads them.
3 Be in touch with your inner self. Then you will be able to understand and to satisfy those physical and psychosocial needs that are important to this final process of writing up your research project.
4 Being in touch with oneself is being reflective and reflexive. Prospective thinkers are those who are always ahead of others in all things that they successfully embark upon. BE THAT PERSON!

Notes

1 Projects are frequently work-based. These are popular with health-related professional courses where there are practical elements to the course.
2 Gantt charts were developed by Henry Gantt, a mechanical engineer, who devised a number of charts for planning and scheduling work (Rouse, 2007).

References

On quality and management

Quality Assurance Agency (2006) *The Code of Practice for the Assurance of Academic Quality and Standards in Higher Education. Section 6: Assessment of Students*. Gloucester: The QAA for Higher Education. Available at: www.qaa.ac.uk/Publications/InformationAndGuidance/Pages/Code-of-practice-Section-6.aspx (accessed 19 January 2012).
Rouse, M. (2007) *What is Gantt Chart?* Search Software Quality at Techtarget website, http://searchsoftwarequality.techtarget.com/definition/Gantt-chart
Stephens, D.C. (ed.) (2000) *The Maslow Business Reader: Abraham H. Maslow*. New York: John Wiley & Sons Inc.

On research and reflection

Coghlan, C. and Pedler, M. (2006) 'Action learning dissertations: structure, supervision and examination', *Action Learning: Research & Practice*, 3(2), 127–139.
Crotty, M. (2003) *The Foundations of Social Research: Meaning and Perspective in Social Research*. London: Sage.
Gibbs, G. (1988) *Learning by Doing: A Guide to Teaching and Learning Methods*. Oxford: Further Education Unit, Oxford Polytechnic.
Johns, C. (2004) *Becoming a Reflective Practitioner* (2nd edn). Oxford: Blackwell.

Redman, P. (2006) *Good Essay Writing: A Social Sciences Guide* (3rd edn). London: Sage.

Schön, D.A. (1991) *The Reflective Practitioner: How Professionals Think in Action.* New York: Basic Books.

Shields, M. (2010) *Essay Writing: A Student's Guide.* Sage Study Skills Series. London: Sage.

On opthalmia neonatorum

Gichuhi, S., Bosire, R., Mbori-Ngacha, D., Gichuhi, C., Wamalwa, D., Maleche-Obimbo, E., Farquhar, C., Wariua, G., Otieno, P. and John-Stewart, G.C. (2009) 'Risk factors for neonatal conjunctivitis in babies of HIV-1 infected mothers', *Ophthalmic Epidemiology*, 16(6), 337–345.

Pilling, R., Long, V., Hobson, R. and Schweiger, M. (2008) 'Opthalmia neonatorum: a vanishing disease or underreported notification? *Eye*, 23, 1879–1880.

Speer, M.E. (2008) 'Gonorrhoea infection in the newborn', *UpToDate*, 19 November, 1–6.

References

Akkerman, S., Admiraal, W., Brekelmans, M. and Oost, H. (2008) 'Auditing quality of research in social sciences', *Quality and Quantitiy*, 42(2), 257–274.

Andrew, S. and Halcomb, E.J. (2009) *Mixed Methods Research for Nursing and the Health Sciences*. Chichester: Wiley-Blackwell.

Anfara, Jr. V.A., Brown, K.M. and Mangione, T.L. (2002) 'Qualitative analysis on stage: making the research process more public', *Educational Researcher*, 31, 28–38. Available at: www.edr.sagepub.com/cgi/content/abstract/31/7/28 (accessed 25 September 2012).

Antman, E.M., Lau, J.M., Kulpenick, B., Mosteller, F. and Chalmers, T.C. (1992) 'A comparison of results of meta-analyses of randomized control trials and recommendations of clinical experts', *Journal of American Medical Association*, 268, 240–245.

Armstrong, E. (2005) *Integrity, Transparency and Accountability in Public Administration: Recent Trends, Regional and International Developments and Emerging Issues*. http:www.upan1.un.org/intradoc/groups/public/.../un/upan020955.pdf

Armstrong, E.R. (2005) *Integrity, Transparency and Accountability in Public Administration: Recent Trends, Regional and International Developments and Emerging Issues*. Economic and Social Affairs, United Nations (www.upan1.un.org/intradoc/groups/public/.../un/unpan020955.pdf).

Auston, I., Cahn, M.A. and Selden, C.R. (1992) *Literature Search Methods for the Development of Clinical Practice Guidelines*. Prepared for the Agency for Health Care Policy and Research, Office of the Forum for Quality and Effectiveness in Health Care, Forum Methodology Conference, 13–16, December. Available at: www.nlm.nih.gov/nichsr/litsrch.html (accessed 29/11/11).

Aveyard, H. (2010) *Doing a Literature Review in Health and Social Care* (2nd edn). Maidenhead: Open University Press.

Barnacle, R. (2005) 'Interpreting interpretation: a phenomenological perspective on phenenography', in J.A. Bowden and P. Green (eds), *Doing Developmental Phenomenography*. Melbourne: RMIT University Press.

Barusch, A., Gringeri, C. and George, M. (2011) 'Rigor in qualitative social work research: a review of strategies used in published articles', *Social Work Research*, 35(1), 11–19.

Beauchamp, T.L. and Childress, J.F. (2008) *Principles of Biomedical Ethics* (6th edn). New York: Oxford University Press.

Bettany-Saltikov, J. (2010) 'Learning how to undertake a systematic literature review: part 1', *Nursing Standard*, 24(50): 47–55.

Blakeman, K. (2012) *Karen Blakeman's Blog*, www.rba.co.uk/wordpress (accessed 09/02/12).

Bluett, E.R. and Cluff, R. (2000) *Principles and Practice of Research in Midwifery*. Edinburgh: Bailliere Tindall.

Boland, R.J., Newman, M. and Pentland, B.T. (2010) 'Hermeneutical exegesis in information system design and use', *Information and Organisation*, 20(1020), 1–20.

Boote, D.N. and Beile, P. (2005) 'Scholars before researchers: on the centrality of the dissertation literature review in research preparation', *Educational Researchers*, 34(6), 3–15.

Booth, A. (2001) 'Cochrane or cock-eyed? How should we conduct systematic reviews of qualitative research?', Paper presented at the Qualitative Evidence-Based Practice Conference, 14–16 May, Coventry University, Coventry, UK. www.leeds.ac.uk/educol/documents/00001724.htm (accessed 27 September 2011).

Boud, D., Keogh, R. and Walker, D. (eds) (1985) *Reflection: Turning Experience into Learning*. New York: Routledge Falmer.

Bowling, A. (2009) *Research Methods in Health: Investigating Health and Health Services* (3rd edn). Maidstone: McGraw-Hill/Open University Press.

Bradbury-Jones, C., Hughes, S.M., Murphy, W., Parry, L. and Sutton, J. (2009) 'A new way of reflecting in nursing: the Peshkin Approach', *Journal of Advanced Nursing*, 65(11), 2485–2493.

Bradley, P. (2011) *Making the Net Easier: Which Search Engine When?*, www.philb.com/whichengine.htm (accessed 01/02/12).

Brannen, J. (2005) 'Mixing methods: the entry of qualitative and quantitative approaches into the research process', *International Journal of Social Research Methodology*, 8(3), 173–184.

Brazier, H. and Begley, C.M. (1996) 'Selecting a database for literature searches in nursing: MEDLINE or CINAHL?', *Journal of Advanced Nursing*, 24(4), 868–875.

Brown, S.J. (2009) *Evidence-Based Nursing: The Research-Practice Connection*. Sudbury, MA: Jones and Bartlett.

Buetow, S. (2010) 'Thematic analysis and its reconceptualisation as "saliency analysis"', *Journal of Health Services Research and Policy*, 15(2), 123–125.

Burns, N. and Grove, S.K. (2001) *The Practice of Nursing Research* (4th edn). Philadelphia, PA: W.B. Saunders.

Burns, N. and Grove, S.K. (2003) *Understanding Nursing Research* (3rd edn). Philadelphia, PA: W.B. Saunders.

Buzan, T. (2002) *How to Mind Map: The Thinking Tool That Will Change Your Mind*. London: Thorsons.

Cambridge Dictionaries (2011) *Cambridge Learner's Dictionary*. Cambridge: Cambridge University Press. Available at: www.dictionary.cambridge.org/dictionary/learner-english (accessed 19/03/12).

Cancer Research UK (2011) Bowel cancer statistics [online] Available at: http://info.cancerresearchuk.org/cancerstats/types/bowel/incidence/uk-bowel-cancer-incidence-statistics [Accessed 13 February 2012].

Carney, T.F. (1990) 'The ladder of analytical abstraction', cited in M.B. Miles and A.M. Huberman (eds) (1994) *Qualitative Data Analysis* (2nd edn). Thousand Oaks, CA: Sage.

Casey, D. and Murphy, K. (2009) 'Issues in using methodological triangulation in research', *Nurse Researcher*, 16(4), 40–55.

Center, M.M., Jemal, A., Smith, R.A. and Ward, E. (2009) 'Worldwide variations in colorectal cancer', *CA: A Cancer Journal for Clinicians*, 59(6), 366–378.

Chalmers, A. (1990) *Science and its Fabrication*. Minneapolis, MN: University of Minnesota Press.

Chalmers, A.F. (2004) *What is This Thing Called Science?* (3rd edn). Milton Keynes: Open University Press.

Chan, L. (2010) 'Body image and the breast: the psychological wound', *Journal of Wound Care*, 19(4), 133–138.

Chapple, A., Ziebland, S., Hewitson, P. and McPherson, A. (2008) 'What affects the uptake of screening for bowel cancer using a faecal occult blood test (FOBt): a qualitative study', *Social Science & Medicine*, 66(12), 2425–2435.

Charmaz, K. (2006) *Constructing Grounded Theory*. Thousand Oaks, CA: Sage.

Cleary-Holdforth, J. and Leufer, T. (2008) 'Essential elements in developing evidence-based practice', *Nursing Standard*, 23(2), 42–46.

Clough, P. and Nutbrown, C. (2000) A Student's Guide to Methodology. London: Sage.

Clyde, A.L. (2005) '*The basis for evidence-based practice: evaluating the research evidence*', *New Library World*, 107(5/6), 180–192. Available at: www.ifla.org/IVfla71/Programee.thm

Coghlan, C. and Pedler, M. (2006) 'Action learning dissertations: structure, supervision and examination', *Action Learning: Research & Practice*, 3(2), 127–139.

Cooper, H. (2010) *Research Meta-Synthesis and Meta-Analysis* (4th edn). Los Angeles: Sage.

Courtney, M. and Jones, J. (2006) 'Impact fever: what is it all about?', *Australian Journal of Advanced Nursing*, 23(4), 6–7.

Crookes, A. and Davies, S. (eds) (2004) Research into Practice (2nd edn). Edinburgh: Bailliere Tindall.

Crotty, M. (2003) *The Foundations of Social Research: Meaning and Perspective in Social Research*. London: Sage.

Davenport, P. (2010) *Report of the Expert Panel on Research Integrity*. Ottawa: Council of Canadian Academies. Available at: www.scienceadvice.ca

De Jonge, A., Teunissen, D.A.M. van Diem, M.Th., Scheepers, P.L.H. and Lagro-Janssen, A.L.M. (2008) 'Women's positions during the second stage of labour: views of primary care midwives', *Journal of Advanced Nursing*, 63(4), 347–356.

Denzin, N.K. and Lincoln, Y.S. (eds) (1998) *Strategies of Qualitative Inquiry*. Thousand Oaks, CA: Sage.

Denzin, N.K. and Lincoln, Y.S. (eds) (2000) *Handbook of Qualitative Research* (2nd edn). London: Sage.

Denzin, N.K. and Lincoln, Y.S. (eds) (2005) *Handbook of Qualitative Research* (3rd edn). London: Sage.

Department of Health (2001) *Research Governance Framework for Health and Social Care*. London: Department of Health.

Depoy, E. and Gitlin, L.N. (2005) *Introduction to Research Understanding and Applying Multiple Strategies* (3rd edn). St Louis, MO: Mosby.

DeSantis, L. and Ugarriza, D.N. (2000) 'The concept of themes as used in qualitative nursing research', *Western Journal of Nursing*, 22, 331.

Descartes, R. (1968) *Discourse on Method and Mediations*. Translated by F.E. Sutcliffe. London: Penguin (originally published 1637).

Dogherty, E., Harrison, M. and Graham, I. (2010) 'Facilitation as a role and process in achieving evidence-based practice in nursing: a focused review of concept and meaning', *Worldview on Evidence-based Nursing, Sigma Theta Tau International Honor Society of Nursing*, 7(2), 76–89.

Doran, G.T. (1981) 'There's a S.M.A.R.T. way to write management goals and objectives', *Management Review*, 70(11), 35–36.

Economic & Social Research Council (2011) *The Research Ethics Guidebook: A Resource for Social Scientist*. Swindon: ESRC. www.ethicsguidebook.ac.uk/Literature-reviews-and-systematuc-reviews-99

Farrell, M.J. and Rose, L. (2008) 'Use of mobile handheld computers in clinical nursing education', *Journal of Nursing Education*, 47(1), 13–19.

Fereday, J., Collins, C., Turnbull, D. and Pincombe, J. (2009) 'An evaluation of midwifery group practice. Part II: women's satisfaction', *Women and Birth*, 22(1), 11–16.

Fleming, S.E. and Vandermause, R. (2011) 'Grand multiparae's evolving experiences of birthing and technology in US hospitals', *Journal of Obstetric, Gynecologic and Neonatal Nursing*, 40(6), 742–752.

Flemming, K. (2007) 'The knowledge base for evidence-based nursing: a role for mixed methods research?', *Advances in Nursing Science*, 30(1), 41–51.

Flick, U. (2009) *An Introduction to Qualitative Research*. London: Sage.

Freeman, B. and Thompson, D. (2009) *Fundamental Aspects of Finding and Using Information: A Guide for Students of Nursing and Health*. London: Quay Books.

Gadamer, H.G. (1984) *Truth and Method*. New York: Crossroads.

Gerrish, K., Guillaume, L., Kirshbaum, M., McDonnell, A. and Nolan, M. (2011) 'Factors influencing the contribution of advanced practice nurses to promote evidence-based practice among front-line nurses: findings from a cross-sectional survey', *Journal of Advanced Nursing*, 67(5), 1079–1090.

Gibbs, G. (1988) *Learning by Doing: A Guide to Teaching and Learning Methods*. Oxford: Further Education Unit, Oxford Polytechnic.

Gichuhi, S., Bosire, R., Mbori-Ngacha, D., Gichuhi, C., Wamalwa, D., Maleche-Obimbo, E., Farquhar, C., Wariua, G., Otieno, P. and John-Stewart, G.C. (2009) 'Risk factors for neonatal conjunctivitis in babies of HIV-1 infected mothers', *Ophthalmic Epidemiology*, 16(6), 337–345.

Glanville, J. (2008) 'Searching shortcuts: finding and appraising search filters', *He@lth Information on the Internet*, 63, 6–8.

Glaser, B.G. (1978) *Theoretical Sensitivity: Advances in the Methodology of Grounded Theory*. Mill Valley, CA: Sociology Press.

Glaser, B.G. (1992) *Emergence vs. Forcing: Basics of Grounded Theory Analysis*. Mill Valley, CA: Sociology Press.

Glaser, B.G. and Strauss, A. (1967) *The Discovery of Grounded Theory*. Chicago, IL: Aldine.

Goodyear, S.J., Leung, E., Menon, A., Pedamallu, S., William, N. and Wong, L.S. (2008) 'The effects of population-based faecal occult blood test screening upon emergency colorectal cancer admissions in Coventry and north Warwickshire', *Gut*, 57, 218–222.

Gorard, S. (2002) 'Can we overcome the methodological schism? Four models for combining qualitative and quantitative evidence', *Research Papers in Education*, 17(4), 345–361.

Gorter, K.J., Tuytel, G.J. and de Leeuw, R.R. (2011) 'Opinions of patients with type 2 diabetes about responsibility, setting targets and willingness to take medication: a cross-sectional survey', *Patient Education and Counselling*, 84(1), 56–61.

Grayling, A.C. (2002) *The Meaning of Things: Applying Philosophy to Life*. London: Phoenix.

Green, B.N., Johnson, C.D. and Adams, A. (2006) 'Writing a narrative literature review for peer-reviewed journal: secret of the trade', *Journal of Chiropractic Medicine*, 5(3), 101–117.

Guba, E.G. (1990) *The Paradigm Dialogue*. London: Sage.

Guba, E.G. and Lincoln, Y.S. (1994) 'Competing paradigms in qualitative research', in N.K. Denzin and Y.S. Lincoln (eds), *Handbook of Qualitative Research*. London: Sage.

Hart, C. (1998) *Doing a Literature Review: Releasing the Social Science Research Imagination*. London: Sage.

Hart, C. (2001) *Doing a Literature Search: A Comprehensive Guide for the Social Sciences*. London: Sage.

Harvey, S., Rach, D., Stainton, M.C., Jarrell, J. and Brant, R. (2002) 'Evaluation of satisfaction with midwifery care', *Midwifery*, 18(4), 260–267.

Hayward, J. (1975) *Information – A Prescription against Pain*. London: Royal College of Nursing.

Hearnshaw, H. and Lindenmeyer, A. (2006) 'What do we mean by adherence to treatment and advice for living with diabetes? A review of the literature on definitions and measurements', *Diabetic Medicine*, 23(7), 720–728.

Higgins, J.P.T. and Green, S. (eds) (2011) *Cochrane Handbook for Systematic Reviews of Interventions Version 5.1.0 [updated March 2011]*. The Cochrane Collaboration. Available at: www.cochrane-handbook.org.

Higgins, P.J. and Green, S. (eds) (2011) *The Cochrane Handbook for Systematic Review of Interventions: The Cochrane Collaboration*. Chichester: John Wiley & Sons Ltd.

Hildingsson, I., Cederlof, L. and Widên, S. (2011) 'Fathers' birth experience in relation to midwifery care', *Women and Birth*, 24(3), 129–136.

Holden, J.D. (2001) 'Hawthorne effects and research into professional practice', *Journal of Evaluation in Clinical Practice*, 7(1), 65–70.

International Journal of Obstetrics and Gynaecology. Available at www.bjog.org/view/0/authorInformation.html

Internet Encyclopaedia of Philosophy (2007) 'Ethics'; *Encyclopaedia of Philosophy* [online] www.iep.utm.edu/e/ethics.htm.

Jarvis, P. (1997) *Ethics and Education for Adults in the Late Modern Society*. Leicester: National Institute of Adult and Continuing Education.

Jarvis, P. (1999) *The Practitioner-Researcher: Developing Theory from Practice*. San Francisco, CA: Jossey-Bass.

Jesson, J., Matheson, L. and Lacey, F.M. (2011) *Doing Your Literature Review: Traditional and Systematic Reviews*. London: Sage.

Johns, C. (2004) *Becoming a Reflective Practitioner* (2nd edn). Oxford: Blackwell.

Journal of Interdisciplinary Health Sciences Author Guidelines: www.hsag.co.za/index.php/HSAG/about/submissions

Koch, T. (2006) 'Establishing rigour in qualitative research: a decision trail', *Journal of Advanced Nursing*, 53(1), 91–103.

Kolb, D.A. (1984) *Experiential Learning: Experience as a Source of Learning and Development*. Upper Saddle River, NJ: Prentice-Hall.

Leininger, M.M. (ed.) (1985) *Qualitative Research Methods in Nursing*. Orlando, FL: Grune and Stratton.

Liberati, A., Altman, D., Tetxlaff, J., Mulrow, C., Gøtzsche, P., Larke, M., Devereaux, P., Kleijnen, J. and Moher, D. (2009) 'The PRISMA statement for reporting systematic reviews and meta-analyses of studies that evaluate health care interventions: explanation and elaboration', *Annals of Internal Medicine*, 151(4), W65–W94.

Lincoln, Y.S. and Guba, E.G. (1985) *Naturalistic Inquiry*. Beverly Hills, CA: Sage.

Lyotard, J. (1984) *The Postmodern Condition: A Report on Knowledge*. Manchester: Manchester University Press.

Machin, A.I., Machin, T. and Pearson, P. (2012) 'Maintaining equilibrium in professional role identity: a grounded theory study of health visitors' perceptions of their changing professional practice context', *Journal of Advanced Nursing*, 68(7), 1526–1537. ncbi.nlm.gov/pubmed/22211526

Marshall, C. and Rossman, G.B. (1995) *Designing Qualitative Research* (2nd edn). Thousand Oaks, CA: Sage.

McCourt, C. (2006) 'Supporting choice and control? Communication and interaction between midwives and women at the antenatal booking visit', *Social Science and Medicine*, 62(6), 1307–1318.

McHenry, L.B. and Jureidini, J.N. (2008) 'Industry-sponsored ghostwriting in clinical trial reporting: a case study', *Accountability in Research*, 15, 152–167.

McQuire, W.J. (1985) 'Attitude and attitude change', cited in G. Lindzey and E. Aronson (eds) (1985) *Handbook of Social Psychology* (3rd edn). New York: Random House.

Medicine Use Review Audit, NHS Leeds 2009–2010 (April 2010). Available at: www.leeds. nhs.uk/About-us/Information%20for%20Professionals/Medicines%20Management/ mur-audit.htm (accessed 5 February 2012)

Mendlinger, S. and Cwikel, J. (2008) 'Spiraling between qualitative and quantitative data on women's health behaviors: a double helix model for mixed methods', *Qualitative Health Research,* 18(2), 280–293.

Mendelson's Theory on Gastric Aspiration (1946): a PatientPlus article (December 2010). Available at: www.patient.co.uk/doctor/Mendelson's-Syndrome.htm (accessed 5 February 2012).

Merriam, S.B. (2001) *Qualitative Research and Case Study Application in Education* (2nd edn). San Francisco, CA: Jossey-Bass.

Meyrick, J. (2006) 'What is good qualitative research? A first step towards a comprehensive approach to judging rigour/quality', *Journal of Health Psychology,* 11(5), 799–808.

Miles, M.B. and Huberman, A.M. (eds) (1994) *Qualitative Data Analysis* (2nd edn). Thousand Oaks, CA: Sage.

Morse, J.M. (ed.) (1994) *Critical Issues in Qualitative Research Methods.* Thousand Oaks, CA: Sage.

Morse, J.M. and Field, P.A. (1995) *Qualitative Research Methods for Health Professionals* (2nd edn). Thousand Oaks, CA: Sage.

Musgrave, A. (1993) *Common Sense, Science and Scepticism: A Historical Introduction to the Theory of Knowledge.* Cambridge: Cambridge University Press.

National Center for Biotechnology Information (2011) *National Library of Medicine Catalog,* www.ncbi.nlm.nih.gov/nlmcatalog (accessed 19/03/12).

Ndosi, M., Vinall, K., Hale, C., Bird, H. and Hill, J. (2011) 'The effectiveness of nurse-led care in people with rheumatoid arthritis: a systematic review', *International Journal of Nursing Studies,* 48(5), 642–654.

NHS Centre for Reviews and Dissemination (2009) *Systematic Reviews: CRD's Guidance for Undertaking Reviews in Health Care.* York: University of York. www.york.ac.uk/inst/crd/ pdf/Systematic_Reviews.pdf (accessed 9 August 2011).

Nursing and Midwifery Council (2008) *The Code: Standards of Conduct, Performance and Ethics for Nurses and Midwives.* London: NMC.

O'Brien, P.M.S. and Pipkin, F.B. (eds) (2007) *Introduction to Research Methodology for Specialists and Trainees* (2nd edn). London: RCOG Press.

O'Donnell, A.B. et al. (2007) 'Using focus group to improve the validity of cross-national survey research: a study of physician decision making', *Qualitative Health Research,* 17(7), 971–981.

Oberle, K. and Allen, M. (2001) 'The nature of advanced practice nursing', *Nursing Outlook,* 49(3), 148–153.

Opler, M.E. (1945) 'Themes as dynamic forces in culture', *American Journal of Sociology,* 51(3), 198–206.

Oxford Dictionaries (1990) *Oxford Dictionary of English.* Oxford: Oxford University Press.

Oxman, A.D. (1994) 'Systematic reviews: checklist for review articles', *British Medical Journal,* 309, 648–661.

Parahoo, K. (2006) *Nursing Research: Principles, Process and Issues* (2nd edn). Basingstoke: Palgrave Macmillan.

Parkin, D.M. (2011a) '5. Cancers attributable to dietary factors in the UK in 2010 – meat consumption', *British Journal of Cancer,* 105, S24–S26.

Parkin, D.M. (2011b) '9. Cancers attributable to inadequate physical exercise in the UK in 2010', *British Journal of Cancer,* 105, S38–S41.

Parkin, D.M. and Boyd, L. (2011a) '4. Cancers attributable to dietary factors in the UK in 2010 – low consumption of fruit and vegetables', *British Journal of Cancer*, 105, S19–S23.

Parkin, D.M. and Boyd, L. (2011b) '6. Cancers attributable to dietary factors in the UK in 2010 – low consumption of fibre', *British Journal of Cancer*, 105, S27–S30.

Parkin, D.M. and Boyd, L. (2011c) '8. Cancers attributable to overweight and obesity in the UK in 2010', *British Journal of Cancer*, 105, S34–S37.

Paterson, B.L., Thorne, S.E., Canam, C. and Jillings, C. (2001) *Meta-Study of Qualitative Health Research: A Practical Guide to Meta-Analysis and Meta-Synthesis.* Thousand Oaks, CA: Sage.

Patton, M. (1990) *Qualitative Evaluation and Research Methods.* Beverly Hills, CA: Sage.

Petticrew, M. and Roberts, H. (2006) *Systematic Reviewing of Literature in the Social Sciences: A Practical Guide.* Oxford: Blackwell.

Pidgeon, N. and Henwood, K. (1996) 'Grounded theory: practical implementation', in J.T.E. Richardson (ed.), *Handbook of Qualitative Research Methods for Psychology and the Social Sciences.* Leicester: BPS Books.

Pilling, R., Long, V., Hobson, R. and Schweiger, M. (2008) 'Opthalmia neonatorum: a vanishing disease or underreported notification? *Eye*, 23, 1879–1880.

Polit, D.F. and Beck, C.T. (2006) *Essentials of Nursing Research: Methods, Appraisal and Utilization* (6th edn). Philadelphia, PA: Lippincott, Williams & Wilkins.

Polit, D.F. and Beck, C.T. (2010) *Essentials of Nursing Research: Appraising Evidence for Nursing Practice* (7th edn). Philadelphia, PA: Wolters Kluwer Health/Lippincott, Williams & Wilkins.

Polit, D.F. and Hungler, B.P. (1999) *Nursing Research: Principles and Methods.* Philadelphia: Lippincott Williams & Wilkins.

Popay, J. (ed.) (2006) *Moving Beyond Effectiveness in Evidence Synthesis: Methodological Issues in the Synthesis of Diverse Sources of Evidence.* London: National Institute for Health and Clinical Excellence (www.nice.org.uk).

Porter, S. (2007) 'Validity, trustworthiness and rigour: reasserting realism in qualitative research', *Journal of Advancing Nursing*, 60(1), 79–86.

Punch, K.F. (2005) *Introduction to Social Research: Quantitative and Qualitative Approaches* (2nd edn). London: Sage.

Punch, K.F. (2003) *Survey Research: The Basics.* London: Sage.

Putnam, J.M. and Riggs, C.J. (2010) 'Involving students in the real world of evidence-based practice', *Journal of Nursing Education*, 49(7), 423–424.

Quality Assurance Agency (2006) *The Code of Practice for the Assurance of Academic Quality and Standards in Higher Education. Section 6: Assessment of Students.* Gloucester: The QAA for Higher Education. Available at: www.qaa.ac.uk/Publications/InformationAndGuidance/Pages/Code-of-practice-Section-6.aspx (accessed 19 January 2012).

Raine, R., Cartwright, M., Richens, Y., Mahamed, Z. and Smith, D. (2010) 'A qualitative study of women's experiences of communication in antenatal care: identifying areas for action', *Maternal and Child Health Journal*, 14(4), 590–599.

Ramberg, B. and Gjesdal, K. (2009) 'Hermeneutics', in N.Z. Edward (eds), *The Stanford Encyclopedia of Philosophy.* Stanford, CA: The Metaphysics Research Lab.

Randolph, J.J. (2009) 'A guide to writing the dissertation literature review', *Practical Assessment, Research and Evaluation*, 14(13), 1–13. www.pareonline.net/getvn.asp?v=14&n=13.

Redman, P. (2006) *Good Essay Writing: A Social Sciences Guide* (3rd edn). London: Sage.

Resnik, D.B. (2011) *What is Ethics in Research and Why is it Important?* Available at: www.niehs.nih.gov/research/resources/bioethics/whatis.cfm (accessed 23 January 2012).

Resnik, D.B. and Master, Z. (2011) 'Authorship policies of bioethics journals', *Journal of Medical Ethics*, 37, 424–428.

Rolfe, G. (2006) 'Validity, trustworthiness and rigour: quality and the idea of qualitative research', *Journal of Advanced Nursing*, 53, 304–310.

Rouse, M. (2007) *What is Gantt Chart?* Search Software Quality at Techtarget website, http://searchsoftwarequality.techtarget.com/definition/Gantt-chart

Royal College of Obstetricians and Gynaecologists (2008) *Standards for Maternity Care: Report of a Working Party*. London: RCOG Press. Available at: www.rcog.org.uk/files/rcog-corp/uploaded-files/WPRMaternityStandards2008.pdf (accessed on 4 July 2012).

Royal College of Obstetricians and Gynaecologists with Royal College of Midwives (2008) *Standards for Maternity Care: Report of a Working Party*. London: RCOG Press. Available at: www.rcog.org.uk/files/rcog-corp/uploaded-files/WPRMaternityStandards2008.pdf.

Ryan, G.W. and Bernard, H.R. (2003) 'Techniques to identify themes', *Field Methods*, 15(1), 85–109.

Sackett, D.L., Richardson, W.S., Rosenberg, W.M.C. and Haynes, R.B. (1997) *Evidence-Based Medicine: How to Practice and Teach EBM*. London: Churchill Livingstone.

Sandelowski, M. (1986) 'The problem of rigor in qualitative research', *Advance Nursing Science*, 8, 27–37.

Sandelowski, M., Barroso, J. and Voils, I.C. (2007) 'Using qualitative metasummary to synthesize qualitative and quantitative descriptive findings', *Research in Nursing and Health*, 30(1), 99–111.

Schön, D.A. (1991) *The Reflective Practitioner: How Professionals Think in Action*. New York: Basic Books.

Scullion, P.A. and Guest, D.A. (2007) *Study Skills for Nursing and Midwifery Students*. Maidenhead: Open University Press.

Sheldon, T.A. (2005) 'Making evidence synthesis more useful for management and policy-making', *Health Service Research Policy*, 10, Supplement 1, 1–15.

Shields, M. (2010) *Essay Writing: A Student's Guide*. Sage Study Skills Series. London: Sage.

Silverman, D. (2010) *Doing Qualitative Research* (3rd edn). London: Sage.

Simon, A.E., Wardle, J. and Miles, A. (2011) 'Is it time to change the stereotype of cancer: the expert view?', *Cancer Causes Control*, 22, 135–140.

Smith, E.R. and Mackie, D.M. (2007) *Social Psychology* (3rd edn). Philadelphia, PA: Psychology Press.

Smith, S. and Bird, D. (2010) 'What do we know already? Searching the literature', in P. Roberts and H. Priest (eds), *Healthcare Research: A Textbook for Students and Practitioners*. Chichester: John Wiley.

Speer, M.E. (2008) 'Gonorrhoea infection in the newborn', *UpToDate*, 19 November, 1–6.

Spradley, J.P. (1979) *The Ethnographic Interview*. New York: Holt, Rhinehart & Winston.

Srivastava, P. and Hopwood, N. (2009) 'A practical iterative framework for qualitative data analysis', *International Journal of Qualitative Methods*, 8(1), 76–84.

Steneck, N.H. (2002) 'Assessing the integrity of publicly supported research', in N.H. Steneck and M.D. Scheetz (eds), *Investigating Research Integrity: Preceedings of the First ORI Research Conference on Research Integrity*. Washington, DC: Office of Research Integrity.

Stephens, D.C. (ed.) (2000) *The Maslow Business Reader: Abraham H. Maslow*. New York: John Wiley & Sons Inc.

Strauss, A. and Corbin, J. (1994) 'Grounded theory methodology: an overview', in N.K. Denzin and Y.S. Lincoln (eds), *Handbook of Qualitative Research*. Thousand Oaks, CA: Sage.

Stremler, R.L. (2003) 'The labour position trial: a randomized, controlled trial of hands and knees positioning for women labouring with a fetus in occipitoposterior position', PhD dissertation, University of Toronto, Toronto (cited in *CINAHL*).

Streubert, H.L. and Carpenter, D.R. (2011) *Qualitative Research in Nursing* (5th edn). Philadelphia, PA: Wolters Kluwer/Lippincott, Williams & Wilkins.

Strike, K. and Posner, G. (1983) 'Types of synthesis and their criteria', in A.W. Spencer and L.J. Reed (eds), *Knowledge, Structure and Use*. Philadelphia, PA: Temple University Press.

Symon, A.G., Dugard, P., Butchart, M., Carr, V. and Paul, J. (2011) 'Care and environment in midwife-led and obstetric-led units: a comparison of mothers' and birth partners' perceptions', *Midwifery*, 27(6), 880–886.

Tashakkori, A. and Teddlie, C. (eds) (2003) *Handbook of Mixed Methods in Social and Behavioural Research*. Thousand Oaks, CA: Sage.

Taylor and Francis Group (2012) *Accountability in Research – Policies and Quality Assurance*. Available at: www.tandf.co.uk/journals/authors/gacraiuth.asp

Taylor-Powell, E. and Renner, M. (2003) *Analyzing Qualitative Data: Programme Development and Evaluation*. Madison: University of Wisconsin-Extension. Available at: www.learningstore. uwex.edu/assets/pdfs/g3658-12.pdf (accessed 4 July 2012).

Teddlie, C.B. and Tashakorri, A. (2009) *Foundations of Mixed Methods Research: Integrating Quantitative and Qualitative Approaches in the Social and Behavioural Sciences*. London: Sage.

UK Legislation (1998) *Data Protection Act*, Chapter 7. London: HMSO.

UK Legislation (2000) *Freedom of Information Act*, Chapter 1. London: HMSO.

von Wagner, C., Good, A., Wright, D., Rachet, B., Obichere, A., Bloom, S. and Wardle, J. (2009) 'Inequalities in colorectal cancer screening participation in the first round of the national screening programme in England', *British Journal of Cancer*, 101, S60–S63.

Waite, M. (ed.) (2009) *Oxford Thesaurus of English* (3rd edn). Oxford: Oxford University Press.

Weed, M. (2005) 'Meta interpretation: a method for the interpretative synthesis of qualitative research', *Forum Qualitative Social Research*, 6(1) [online article], www.qualitative-research.net/index.php/fqs/article/view/508/1096 (accessed 9 February 2012).

Willis, J.W. (2007) *Foundations of Qualitative Research*. Thousand Oaks, CA: Sage.

Whittemore, R. and Knafl, K. (2005) 'The integrative review: updated methodology', *Journal of Advanced Nursing*, 52(5), 546–553.

Yin, R.K. (2003) *Case Study Research: Design and Methods* (3rd edn). London: Sage.

Index

data analysis
  evaluation of 106, 107
  process 59–60
data collection
  appropriateness to sample size and
    sampling type 104–105
  evaluation of 103–105
  process 58–59
data convergence 146, 148, 149
data extraction summary table 125,
  128–129, 140
data extraction tool 61, 95
data protection act 14
databases
  bibliographic 74–76
  citation 76
  full-text 76
  search engines 76–77
deductive paradigm 6, 8–9, 40
defining scope of research topic 36–38
  clients' perspectives 36–37
  colleagues' perspectives 36–37
  exploring the literature 37–38
  key words 38, 67–68
  number of studies to review 38
  personal experience 34–35, 38
  practice setting 34–35
  search engines 68
degree classification 161
development of categories 130–131,
  132–133, 135–136
development of themes 123–137, 145,
  147, 169
  analysis stage 123, 127–131
  exploratory stage 123, 124–127
  synthesis stage 123
Diabetes adherence 38, 59
discussion and conclusion
  (evaluation of) 108
dissertation 74

E

empirical and non-empirical research
  13–16
  philosophical basis 45
  processes compared 16–17, 18–19

EndNote or reference management
  software 85, 171
Epistemology 25–26, 30, 32
  definition 28
ethical considerations of research 60,
  62–63
  conduct and misconduct 88–89
ethical principle of accountability in
  comprehensive literature review 63,
  93–95, 110, 113, 131, 145, 150
  actions 94–95
  decisions 94
  impact on client care 94–95
ethical principle of integrity in
  comprehensive literature review 63,
  90–92, 110, 113, 131, 145, 150
  fairness 92
  honesty 91
  truthfulness 92
ethical principle of transparency in
  comprehensive literature review
  63, 92–93, 110, 113, 131, 145, 150
  accessibility 93
  accuracy 93
  openness 93
Ethics (definitions) 62
evaluative criteria for comprehensive
  literature review 95–108
  author/researcher 97
  source of publication 96–97
  title of paper 97
everyday life world and professional
  world 26
evidence-based healthcare 5
evidence-based practice 156
exploratory stage in theme
  development 123, 124–127

F

findings (evaluation of) 106–107
  mixed methodology: balanced
    presentation 107
  qualitative research: rich description
    106–107
  quantitative research: diagrammatic
    representation 106–107

findings (of your research project)
  discussing 144–153
  disseminating 155–156
  justifying 152–153
  presenting (suggested format) 141
  summary of grey literature 144
  summary of qualitative
    research 143
  summary of quantitative
    research 142
Freedom of information act 14
fusion of horizons 134–137

G

Gantt chart 114, 162, 173, 174
grey literature 74
  evaluative criteria 108–110
  types 55

H

helical process 67
hermeneutic exegesis 115, 118–120,
    124, 134
  characteristics (4 criteria) 118–119
hermeneutic process 95

I

identifying research topic 33–36
  clients' perspectives 36–37
  colleagues' perspectives 36–37
  exploring the literature 37–38
  key words 38
  number of studies to review 38
  personal experience 34–35, 38
  practice setting 34–35
implications of your research project
    findings 155–156
inclusion and exclusion criteria in
    sampling 58
inductive paradigm 6, 7–8, 40
interpretivism 6, 7, 31, 32, 33, 53
interpretivist school of thought
    30–33
inter-rater reliability 105

inverted comas in searching 84
iterative process 52, 67, 116, 120, 131

J

journal article search 74–77

K

keywords 67–69, 78–80, 83
  spelling 79
  truncation symbols 79–80
  wildcard 79–80
knowledge
  continuum (novice to expert) 4
  general and particular 3–4
  meaning 2
  roots 23
  scope 22–25
  sources 3–4

L

labour positions 8, 29, 69, 80–81
library catalogues 73
literature
  empirical and non-empirical 37
literature review 41
  currency or datedness of literature
    (evaluation of) 98–99
  preliminary (evaluation of) 98–99
literature review methodology 13–14,
    15–16, 46
  characteristics 14, 46
  definition 15
  process 16–17
  types 46–47
literature search(es)
  log or record of 59, 85
  pararmeters 69–72, 77, 85
  preliminary 67

M

marking criteria 161, 171–172
merits and flaws of research literature
    146–147